Medicine's 10 Greatest Discoveries

Meyer Friedman, M.D.
Gerald W. Friedland, M.D.

Medicine's

10

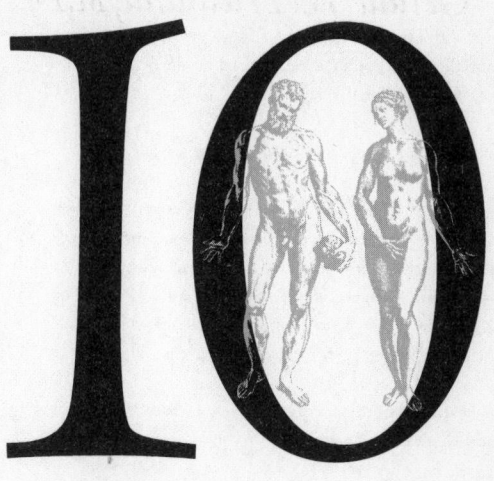

Greatest

Discoveries

Yale Nota Bene

Yale University Press

New Haven & London

Published with assistance from the Kingsley Trust
Association Publication Fund established by the Scroll
and Key Society of Yale College.

First published as a Yale Nota Bene book in 2000.

For information about this and other Yale University Press
publications, please contact:
    U.S. office   sales.press@yale.edu
    Europe office   sales@yaleup.co.uk

Printed in the United States of America.

The Library of Congress has cataloged the hardcover
edition as follows:
    Friedman, Meyer, 1910–
    Medicine's 10 greatest discoveries / Meyer Friedman, and
    Gerald W. Friedland.
        p.   cm.
    Includes bibliographical references and index.
    ISBN 0-300-07598-7 (cloth : alk. paper)
    1. Medicine—History. 2. Medical scientists. I. Friedland,
    Gerald W.
    R145. F75   1998
    610'.9—dc21   98–19921

ISBN 0-300-08278-9 (pbk.)

A catalogue record for this book is available from the British Library.

10 9 8 7 6 5 4 3

To our physician-wives,
Macia Campbell Friedman (deceased)
and Miriam Friedland

Contents

Preface

This book does not describe the history or the evolution of Western medicine. Many fine accounts of these matters are already available. Nor does this book list all the great medical discoveries since Andreas Vesalius in 1543 awakened the medical world from fourteen centuries of torpor with the publication of his astonishing book *De humani corporis fabrica, libri septem,* usually referred to as the *Fabrica.*

What this book does dare to do is select and describe what we consider to be the ten most significant medical discoveries since 1543. Without these indispensable plinths, medicine as we know and practice it today would not be possible. Our volume also gives an intimate account of the lives of the scientists principally responsible for the ten transcendent discoveries.

In the title of each of the chapters describing these ten discoveries is the name of the person who we believe began the process of discovery. But we also recount the later contributions of other researchers who continued that process. Thus, we feature Antony Leeuwenhoek in the chapter dealing with bacteria, but we also present the magnificent work of Robert Koch, Louis Pasteur, and others. Similarly, in the chapter treating the discovery of antibiotics, it is Alexander Fleming who appears in the chapter title; but we have not forgotten the awesome contributions of researchers such as Howard Florey and Ernst Chain.

For whom have we written this book? Certainly any reasonably intelligent and moderately educated adult who is even slightly interested in medicine should find this book pleasing, even absorbing. High school and college students drawn to science and medicine may find the chapters exciting. Physicians will surely discern much that is new to them and, we hope, enjoyable. Wistfully, we wish that medical students, interns, and residents could find the time to peruse this book. Were they to do so, we are positive that their time would not be wasted. And if readers experience even a fraction of our own joy and fascination in ferreting out facts and incidents, our pleasurable labors will not have been in vain.

In relating the history of these discoveries, we have tried insofar as possible to avoid medical jargon. But because we aim to inform the physician as well as the lay reader, we have accompanied our descriptions with notes that strive to amplify but not distract.

Our readers have a right to know something about the construction of this book. They may wonder whether the authors are qualified to make these selections, and they may be curious about the criteria employed in singling out medicine's ten most dazzling accomplishments.

One of us has spent forty-six years, the other sixty-six years, in studying, practicing, and teaching medicine to medical students. Both of us have spent decades ourselves in making medical discoveries. We have published well over five hundred medical articles and a half-dozen medical books. So, after a combined total of one hundred twelve years of such activity, we believe we are familiar with most of the major discoveries of medicine and should be able to choose the ten that are of surpassing importance.

As to the criteria employed in selecting the ten ultimate discoveries, we first surveyed the three components of the field of medicine: the structures and functions of the human body and mind, the diagnosis of medical disorders and injuries, and the treatment of such maladies. We asked ourselves which ten discoveries, of the thousands that have been made, tower above all others in these three areas.

Relatively easily, we selected what we considered to be the hundred most significant discoveries of the five thousand or more that have been made in Western medicine. Our task became more difficult when we tried to narrow our selection to twenty-five. For example, the unearthing of both surgical antisepsis and asepsis to prevent bacterial infection in surgical wounds was significant indeed, but Koch's finding that bacteria were the cause of infection was even more important. Again, the discoveries of insulin and cortisone (both of which won a Nobel Prize) were on our preliminary list of one hundred; crucial as both were, the detection of bacteria and the development of anesthesia had vastly more repercussions.

After we had finally selected the ten breakthroughs described in this book, we presented our list to three antiquarian medical book dealers whose commercial success depends on their knowledge of the comparative significance of medical discoveries. For example, the findings of men such as Fracastorius, Auenbrügger, and Servetus, which are not known to most physicians, are as familiar to antiquarian booksellers as the letters of the English alphabet. Further, these dealers know well enough that an offprint of the first description of the discovery of cortisone is as rare as an offprint of the first description of the structure of DNA. They would pay only several hundred dollars for the cortisone offprint, but well over $25,000 for the DNA offprint—a monetary difference due solely to their relative medical importance.

Our list of ten was presented next to four avid and informed physician-collectors of rare and important medical publications, including first editions of the published descriptions of most of the advances in this book. All agreed that our ten ranked as the major breakthroughs of Western medicine.

After these preliminary samplings, we individually asked thirty or more physicians affiliated with either Stanford University or the University of California Medical School if they could identify the investigators responsible for the ten discoveries we had selected. All were able to identify Andreas Vesalius, William Harvey, Edward Jenner, Wilhelm Roentgen, Alexander Fleming, James Watson, and Francis Crick. Most also had a vague recollection of Antony Leeuwenhoek as a microscopist, but not as the discoverer of bacteria. None of these physicians, who teach medical students, interns, and residents, were aware of Ross Harrison, Nicholai Anichkov, or Maurice Wilkins. Only two were able to identify Crawford Long. However, when we enumerated the ten discoveries we considered the most important, and our reasons for nominating them, all but one physician agreed with our choices. Nevertheless, we were surprised that so many of the doctors we interviewed knew so little about the lives and achievements of their great predecessors.

Interestingly, too, when we inquired of the presidents of Johns Hopkins and Yale universities whether either university had a memorial commemorating the Ross Harrison invention of tissue culture, neither was able to recall who Harrison was. But Harrison published his preliminary paper on this procedure in 1907, while still at Hopkins, and a final and complete article appeared in 1910 while he was at Yale. (Later, the president of Yale wrote to tell us that a professorial chair has been established at Yale in Harrison's honor. And the president of Johns Hopkins informed us that a photograph of Harrison is now on display in the lobby of the Johns Hopkins hospital.)

Three of the eleven chapters in this book deal with discoveries concerning the structures and functions of the normal human body and mind. Six chapters describe findings relative to the treatment of medical disorders and injuries. The remaining chapter tells of the accidental discovery of medicine's principal diagnostic tool, the X-ray machine, and the subsequent fabrication of the computerized tomographic (CT) scanner.

In our final chapter, we single out what we consider the apogee of all the medical discoveries. As readers peruse our chapters, in which the ten discoveries are presented in chronological order, they may be interested in choosing their own "single most important discovery." We invite a comparison of that selection with ours, which we reveal in Chapter 11.

Major components of this book could not have been written without the data kindly provided us by a number of distinguished scientists, and we thank all of them:

Nobel laureates Godfrey Hounsfield and Allan Cormack, as well as Dr. James Ambrose responded to our questions as we prepared Chapter 6.

Professors Leonard Hayflick, Sergey Federoff, and Richard Hamm, and Doctors George Farell, Donna Peehl, Robert Stevenson, and Elizabeth Harrison (the ninety-eight-year-old daughter of Ross Harrison) graciously provided historical facts for the writing of Chapter 7.

Nobel laureates Frances Crick, Sir Aaron Klug, Sir Peter Medawar, James Watson, and Maurice Wilkins, and Professors Erwin Chargaff and Raymond Gosling, together with Jane Callander (formerly with the British Broadcasting Company), granted us numerous interviews that were indispensable to the construction of Chapter 10.

We are especially grateful to Robert Schindler, chairman of the Department of Otolaryngology of the University of California, San Francisco, who was instrumental in the preliminary selection of the hundred greatest discoveries, which we eventually narrowed to the ten described herein.

We express our thanks to Ranny Riley, who first suggested that a book of this sort might be of general interest to the reading public.

We are deeply indebted to Linda Ball, Kevin Murphy, Diane Remillard, and Jean Chan, who were responsible for the typing of the manuscript and the development of the photographs.

Finally, we are grateful for the continuing advice given us by James C. Nelson, Dr. Barton Sparagon, and Professor Barton Thurber, as well as the editorial services given by Vivian B. Wheeler.

Medicine's 10 Greatest Discoveries

I

Andreas Vesalius and

Modern Human Anatomy

We give full credit in this chapter to Andreas Vesalius for the first great discovery of Western medicine, but he had precursors, and we need to look first at their achievements.

Although Hippocrates and Aristotle were vaguely knowledgeable about some of the bones and muscles of the human body, neither had ever dissected a human body. What little information they had about human organs was derived from their dissection of animals. However, Herophilus of Alexandria in the fourth century B.C. was able to dissect some human corpses. The observations he derived from these dissections, had they not been destroyed by fire, would have done much to prevent the nineteen centuries of almost total anatomical dubiety that prevailed from his time to the era of Vesalius. But the loss of Herophilus' anatomical observations was only one of the reasons why anatomy failed to flourish as a branch of medical knowledge.

Another major reason was the writings of Galen, a Greek physician of the second century A.D. His anatomical observations took on, for many centuries, a Christian sacredness so fervent that to criticize any of them was life-endangering heresy. Yet many of the supposedly human organs he described actually derived from his observations of dogs or apes, as Galen himself admitted. Apparently even in Roman times, human dissection was forbidden.

Another reason for the failure of an anatomical science to begin before the Renaissance was the strange (to us) lethargy that captured the medieval mind. Seemingly no one cared much about intellectual, artistic, or scientific activity. It was as if the survivors of the dying Roman Empire were exhausted from its stresses. As century after century went by, only the scribblings of cloistered monks preserved the Latin language, a few fragments of Greek and Roman literature, and the Bible. All else characterizing a fully alive civilization disappeared until the long torpor gradually gave way to the slow awakening we now designate as the Renaissance. We shall never quite understand why Western civilization could sleep for so many centuries or why it finally awakened.

A fourth reason for the failure of the science of anatomy to develop was the almost universal prohibition of dissection of human bodies. Again, it was not until the start of the Renaissance that a few Italian city-states (notably Bologna, Padua, and Pavia) began to permit the dissection of a few executed felons each year. In a sense, it was these dead criminals who gave birth to modern anatomy.

Mondino DeLuzzi of Bologna, in his *Anothomia* (written in 1316 but not printed until 1478),[1] was the first to perform and describe dissections of the human body. However, the "sacred" but erroneous anatomical observations of Galen so blinded Mondino that he was unable to see what stared up at him. Like Galen more than a thousand years earlier, Mondino wrongly described the spleen as emptying into the stomach, the liver as five-lobed, the heart as possessed of three ventricles, and the uterus as composed of multiple segments. Some of his writings may have accurately depicted the organs of a dog, but not of a man or a woman. Yet DeLuzzi's *Anothomia*, published in more than sixty editions, served for two hundred years as the chief source of understanding of human gross anatomy.

In 1521 Berengario da Carpi, incumbent of the chair of surgery and anatomy at Bologna, after reportedly dissecting more than a hundred human bodies published his *Commentaries* on the *Anothomia*. This book, more than a thousand pages in length, for the first time carried anatomical illustrations—although they were little more than crude diagrams. More important, da Carpi dared for the first time in medieval and early Renaissance history, to correct some of Galen's more egregious anatomical misconceptions. No longer was the heart depicted as having three ventricles or the uterus as being multisegmented, as they had been erroneously described for fourteen centuries. The science of human anatomy was about to be born.

We know when and where Vesalius was born (1514 in Brussels), what universities he attended (Louvain, Paris, and Padua), and when and where he received his medical degree (1537 from Padua). We even know whom and when he married (Anne van Hamme in 1544) and that he had one daughter (Anne). We know that in 1546 he became a court physician to the Holy Roman Emperor Charles V and remained in imperial service until Charles's abdication in 1556, after which Vesalius attended Philip II, king of Spain. He continued in royal service until he died in 1564 on his return from a pilgrimage to Jerusalem.

No one knows exactly why Vesalius made this hazardous voyage—perhaps as penance for some dreadful mistake. One persistent rumor is that he began to dissect a supposedly dead nobleman whose heart was found to be still beating. For this grisly error he was sentenced to death by the Inquisition authorities, but King Philip substituted the pilgrimage for his decreed execution. Whatever the true reason, it is virtually certain that Vesalius did not make this pilgrimage because of his spiritual convictions.

We would not have known (or cared to know) these skimpy details of Vesalius' life had he not in 1543 published a book described by William Osler, the father of American medicine, as "the greatest book in medicine." Before we assess this revolutionary and supremely elegant volume, let us examine the personality of the high Renaissance physician who wrote it and the sort of life he experienced. We get some idea of his character when we read that at age thirty-two he looked back at his younger self and described certain pursuits in which he once indulged but which he no longer wished to perpetuate.[2]

At present I shouldn't willingly spend long hours in the Cemetery of the Innocents in Paris turning over bones nor go to Montfaucon to look for bones—when once with a companion, I was gravely imperiled by many savage dogs. Nor should I care to be locked out of Louvain [University] so that, alone in the middle of the night, I might take away bones from the gibbet to prepare a skeleton. I shall no longer bother to petition the judges to delay the day of an execution of a criminal to a time suitable for my dissection of his body nor shall I advise the medical students to observe where someone has been buried or urge them to make note of the diseases of their teachers' patients so that they might later seize their bodies. I shall not keep in my bedroom for several weeks bodies taken from graves or given me after public execution, nor shall I put up with the bad temper of sculptors and painters who made me more miserable than did the bodies I was dissecting. However too young to gain financially from the art and wishing to learn and to advance our common studies, I readily and cheerfully supported all these things.

This horrendous account of his activities, first as a medical student in Paris and later as an anatomist in Padua, reveals a young Vesalius who was fanatically determined, whatever the cost, to learn the secrets of the human body. He savaged corpses for their bones and competed with ferocious dogs for their flesh. What can we say about a man who encouraged his medical students to record their teachers' sick patients in order to steal the corpses when the patients died? What sort of man can sleep night after night with rotting bodies in his bedroom? And how meticulously demanding must have been his dealings with sculptors and painters so that they would depict a tissue or an organ exactly as he viewed it at the dissecting table! By no standard could Vesalius be considered either charming or compassionate. He was primarily a cold-hearted, determined, extraordinarily ambitious man.

When he went to Paris in 1533 to continue his medical studies, he was only nineteen years old and already had set his mind on becoming so distinguished a surgeon and anatomist that he would be appointed by Emperor Charles V as one of his physicians. After all, his grandfather and his father, too (despite his father's illegitimacy), had entered the imperial service.

With such aspirations, the Flemish youth became so adept at dissecting animals that he attracted the attention of the two most famous anatomists of Europe, Jacob Sylvius and John Guinter, both of whom were teaching at the University of Paris. Sylvius taught Vesalius how to dissect dogs, whereas Guinter used him as an assistant in his dissection of human corpses. This was the period during which Vesalius, on his own, frequented Parisian cemeteries in order to gather human bones.

In 1536 Vesalius, as a Fleming and a loyal subject of Charles V, had to leave Paris because of the grave danger that this Holy Roman Emperor might invade Paris. Returning to Brussels, Vesalius continued his medical career at Louvain University. Already he was secretly dissecting human bodies.

He left Louvain in 1539 for the University of Padua, where he received his degree in medicine a few months after his arrival. He was so learned and skilled in dissection of human corpses that several weeks after he received his medical degree, at the young age of twenty-three years, he was appointed head of the Department of Surgery and Anatomy at Padua. He continued to dissect the corpses of both animals and executed criminals — and surreptitiously others stolen from cemeteries.

Like all anatomists for centuries before him, for several years Vesalius continued to construe the human body as Galen had described it rather than acknowledging what his own eyes discerned. But in 1538 he published *Tabulae anatomicae sex*,[3] in which he first dared to point out several errors that Galen had made. Admittedly they were relatively small mistakes, but no anatomist for fourteen centuries had dared to correct them. Even more startling, this same publication, for the first time in the five centuries of recorded medical writings, carried six illustrations that were not crude cartoons but artistically fetching, realistic representations of human bones and muscles.[4]

There is no question that the illustrator who drew the last three drawings in the *Tabulae* was a painter in Titian's studio, one John Stephanus of Calcar. Actually this painter paid for the printing of the book and received whatever profit it brought in. Just why this peculiar financial arrangement was made we shall never know. Nor shall we ever discover precisely what sort of man Stephanus was.

Vesalius, even before publication of the *Tabulae*, differed from his predecessors and his contemporaries, who were accustomed to sitting on a chair far above the body being dissected by a barber, reading a Galenical textbook to their students, and paying no attention whatsoever to the tissues and organs of the body beneath them. Instead, Vesalius himself dissected the corpse, bloodying his hands and his clothes as he handled these often infected and putrefying organs. It was his fervent belief that for a person to know the human body, that person must dissect it. He never tired of preaching this pedagogical concept to his medical students and the physician-colleagues who attended his public dissections.

However, in the sixteenth century during which he was dirtying and contaminating his hands, and possibly also his face, protective gloves and antiseptics did not yet exist. Even worse, there was absolutely no awareness of the existence of bacteria or viruses and the lethal diseases they caused. So it is no wonder that Vesalius and his three most talented students (Columbus, Eustachius, and Fallopius)—as eager as Vesalius to contaminate their hands with the tissues even of infected bodies—all died before the age of fifty-five. In marked contrast, four artists (Michelangelo, Leonardo, Titian, and Cellini) of the same period and the same cities all lived beyond their sixty-fifth birthday and two of them (Michelangelo and Titian) past their eighty-fifth birthday. It would seem that at this time it was far more perilous to dissect flesh than to paint or sculpt it.

Following publication of the *Tabulae*, Vesalius' further writings until 1543 were of little consequence. He continued to dissect bodies and teach medical students at Padua, and for a short while also at Bologna. Even at the young age of twenty-nine years—at which time his *Fabrica* appeared [5]—he was esteemed in Italy, Paris, and Brussels as an anatomist who was marvelously adept at the dissection of human bodies.

Then in 1544, one year after he published the *Fabrica*, he left the University of Padua and entered the imperial court of Charles V as one of the emperor's physicians. Some medical historians have been shocked and puzzled at this seemingly abrupt termination of his academic career. But imperial service, as we have already emphasized, was the ultimate goal of the ambitious and totally pragmatic Vesalius. No one ever accused him of any nimiety of loyalty to a university or medical school. Such nicety of feeling could not be possessed by a man who in the dead of night vied in cemeteries with packs of hungry dogs for barely covered corpses, a man who could calmly, cruelly, vivisect animals despite their heart-rending shrieks of pain.

We have mentioned that Vesalius in 1544 married Anne van Hamme of Brussels, who gave birth the following year to a daughter, also named Anne. We know almost nothing about wife or daughter, except that both of them married one year after he died. Suspicion exists that his relationship with both was less than endearing.

His lifelong ambition to enter the imperial medical service fulfilled, Vesalius totally ceased all scientific studies. Yet he was esteemed throughout Europe as one of its most capable physicians. In 1559 when Henry II, king of France, was gravely injured in a jousting contest, Vesalius was summoned from Brussels to Paris to attend him. Henry II (perhaps best remembered today because of the transcendent beauty of his mistress, Diane de Poitiers, and the enduring courage and cunning of his wife, Catherine de Medici) had received a blow to the face and head from the splinters of a lance that ruptured as it pierced his helmet. Prior to Vesalius' arrival, Henry's physicians had been unable to determine exactly how far the splinters had pierced his head. They obtained the stump of the splintered lance and jammed it with great force into the heads of four decapitated criminals, who had been executed the day before. The physicians then dissected each head to determine whether any of the splinters had entered the brain. This extraordinary "experiment" proved useless.

Vesalius, after examining the stricken king, knew and announced that the injury would be fatal. Despite frequent venesections and purges, the king suffered complete paralysis on the left side of his body and convulsions on the right side, and died approximately ten days later. Vesalius attended the autopsy, which revealed severe brain injury and a subdural hemorrhage over the right side of his brain.

In another show of confidence in Vesalius' abilities, when Don Carlos, crown prince of Spain, became gravely ill in 1562, Vesalius was dispatched by Philip II to oversee the five other physicians already in attendance. This illness had also begun with an injury.

Don Carlos—short, cruel, and stubborn—even at his birth had been a problem to his father, Philip II. Born with teeth, as a suckling baby Don Carlos chewed so viciously on the nipples of the women nursing him that their breasts were mangled and became infected. At twelve years of age, he had two preoccupations: roasting animals alive and seducing pretty girls.

It was the second obsession that was responsible for his injury in early April of his eighteenth year. Spotting the caretaker's daughter (with whom he was infatuated) walking outside in the garden, he became so excited running down the steps to meet her that he stumbled and turned a complete somersault. His head hit the knob of a door at the foot of the stairs. Although he recovered consciousness rapidly enough, the three attending physicians found that he had sustained a thumbnail-sized contusion at the back of his neck. The wound was elaborately dressed with liquids and ointments of various kinds. As was the custom, he was both bled and purged.

Probably because of the unsterile dressings applied to his wound, it festered. The prince became quite feverish. Philip II, alarmed, sent two of his own royal physicians to join the three physicians already in attendance on Don Carlos. When his son's condition continued to worsen, he sent for Vesalius to take charge.

The six physicians held fifty consultations, ten of which were attended by the king. He patiently listened for two to four hours, during which each physician gave his opinion of what should be done. The condition of Don Carlos, despite these multiple consultations, steadily worsened throughout April and May.

Meanwhile, three thousand Spaniards at Toledo, stripped to the waist, paraded as they scourged each other, hoping that such flagellation might save the prince's life. In contrast, the citizens of Alcala (where the prince lay apparently dying) carried the mummified corpse of Fra Diego, a Franciscan friar who had died several centuries earlier, to the bed of Don Carlos and placed it next to the body of the unconscious prince.

No numinous medical miracle instantly took place, but in the days and weeks that elapsed, the prince recovered from his fever and delirium. His infected face, which had been distorted by hemorrhage and accumulation of pus, gradually recovered its usual form. Three months after becoming ill, he had recovered sufficiently to attend a bullfight.

Philip II always thought that it was the mummified corpse of Fra Diego that had eventually cured his son. He saw to it in 1568 that the Franciscan monk was sanctified. Whether Philip was correct in this belief we cannot be sure. But we *can* be sure that every deadly complication ensuing after Don Carlos' simple concussion was of iatrogenic origin.

These two royal consultative involvements are the only items history records of Vesalius' twenty years of imperial service—except for his *Letter on the China Root*, published by his younger brother in 1546; his second edition in 1555 of the *Fabrica*; and his comments (the *Examen*) in 1561 on the "anatomical observations" of his former student Fallopius. None of these publications presented the results of any new studies. Again, we question why this young man—after publishing a book (the *Fabrica*) whose contents essentially gave birth to modern scientific medicine—should at the age of twenty-nine cease performing scientific or medical studies of any kind.

He himself wrote in 1546, three years after publication of the *Fabrica*, that this book evoked so many unfounded criticisms that "gnawed at his soul" that he escaped to the imperial court, content to live there "far from the sweet leisure of studies . . . . Thus I would not consider publishing anything new even if I wanted to do so very much or if my vanity urged me to do it."[6]

Vesalius from the outset of his career hoped and schemed to be invited by the emperor to join his cadre of imperial physicians. The young author in 1537, when he was only twenty-three years of age, planned to write and publish a book that would be not only revolutionary in content but also elegant in typography, paper, illustrations, size, and binding. The emperor, although unversed in medicine, would recognize that this book, dedicated to him and personally presented to him by Vesalius, was and forever would be the most dazzling book of medicine ever printed.

Sure enough, as Vesalius himself wrote, unhampered by a wife, children, or domestic cares, he devoted probably five years to dissecting dozens of corpses of humans and animals—to gain the encyclopedic knowledge he needed for the text of this book. He also had to find artists willing to spend hours making sketches of the organs and tissues of decaying bodies. His book, the *Fabrica*, would be the first medical book in history to carry stunning illustrations, well over two hundred of them.

Vesalius even had the courage to send his manuscript across the Alps to Basel. He knew that there John Oporinus, a distinguished professor and, more important, a superb printer, would grant his book the finest paper and the most exquisite printing possible. Vesalius, above all, was certain that Oporinus had the skill to print his precious woodcut engravings with the delicate, precise accuracy he desired. Not content with merely sending letters of detailed instructions to Oporinus, Vesalius journeyed to Basel and remained there while the book was being printed.

In the late summer of 1543, Vesalius presented his masterpiece to Charles V. And masterpiece it was, with its height of 16.5 inches, its width of 11 inches, its binding of imperial purple silk velvet, its front and back leaves of vellum, and its *seven hundred* pages displaying the finest typography ever seen in a medical book. The spectacular glory of this presentation copy was its *hand-colored* illustrations. (None of the hundred or so extant copies has any colored illustrations.) The emperor must have been enormously impressed. It was no surprise that a few months later, despite the envious criticism of his work by other physicians attending the emperor, Vesalius was invited into the imperial service. His young life's ambition had been realized.

Now it is appropriate that we turn our attention to his immortal masterpiece: *De humani corporis fabrica, libri septem,* usually referred to as the *Fabrica*.

While medical scholars might be hesitant to agree that this revelation of the anatomy of the human body in seven books (as its Latin title declares) is the most important discovery in Western medicine, certainly all would agree with William Osler that *Fabrica* is the greatest medical book ever to appear.

We have already intimated that it was Vesalius' intent to dedicate, and then present, to Charles V a book that would overwhelm him with its magnificence and elegance. But this *Fabrica* did far more than merely charm an emperor—who after all could not understand or appreciate the content of the book. Its appearance awakened medicine from fourteen centuries of very deep sleep.

The first reaction of physicians to the appearance of the *Fabrica* was one of amazement. Never before had a medical book possessed such height and width. Never before had a medical book contained illustrations of such artistic beauty and anatomical precision, and never before (or since) had a medical book been published with such elegant typography.

Most of Vesalius' medical colleagues at first were astounded at the sheer tastefulness and sumptuousness of the *Fabrica*. But the text filling the seven books shocked many of his contemporaries and infuriated quite a few of them. So maddened was Jacob Sylvius, Vesalius' former anatomy teacher and the foremost anatomist of Europe, that in an open letter to the emperor, he wrote: "I implore His Imperial Majesty to punish severely, as he deserves, this monster born and bred in his own house, this worst example of ignorance, ingratitude, arrogance, and impiety, to suppress him so that he may not poison the rest of Europe with his pestilential breath."

Sylvius' anger was fueled by the fact that Vesalius had dared to point out Galen's repeated errors in describing certain aspects of human anatomy, primarily because he had dissected and hence described the tissues and organs of monkeys and dogs, not of human beings.

Why such fury, when dissections of human bodies in the late Middle Ages had revealed the absurdities of some of Galen's observations; for instance, that the liver gave rise to blood, that the uterus had multiple chambers, and that the pituitary poured its secretions directly into the nose? We have seen that no medical professor ever dissected human bodies. The dissection was done by a barber, while the professor read aloud from one of Galen's books of anatomical observations. This centuries-old custom died within a decade of the publication of the *Fabrica*. Indeed, a fair portion of the book was devoted to specific instructions on how to dissect a corpse.

The *Fabrica* also emphasized a fact that heretofore had been overlooked: namely, that the bones of the body made possible life as we know it. The book pointed out that our bones not only give support and mobility to the rest of our body, but they also protect our frail organs (including the brain) from injury. Vesalius emphasized that were it not for our bones, we would be immobile structural blobs.

It is immediately apparent on perusing the *Fabrica* that Vesalius was totally fascinated with human bones. In the first of the seven books, he devotes 168 pages to them. In a burst of pictorial splendor, he begins Book 1 with a display of five skulls viewed from different angles. He then describes and portrays, in superb sketches, the remaining bones of the body. In an amazing tour de force, he ends Book 1 with three full-page drawings of complete skeletons. One appears suspended from a gibbet, another appears to be striding with the aid of a crutch, and the third (see Fig. 1), elbows leaning on a desk, appears to be contemplating the interior of a human

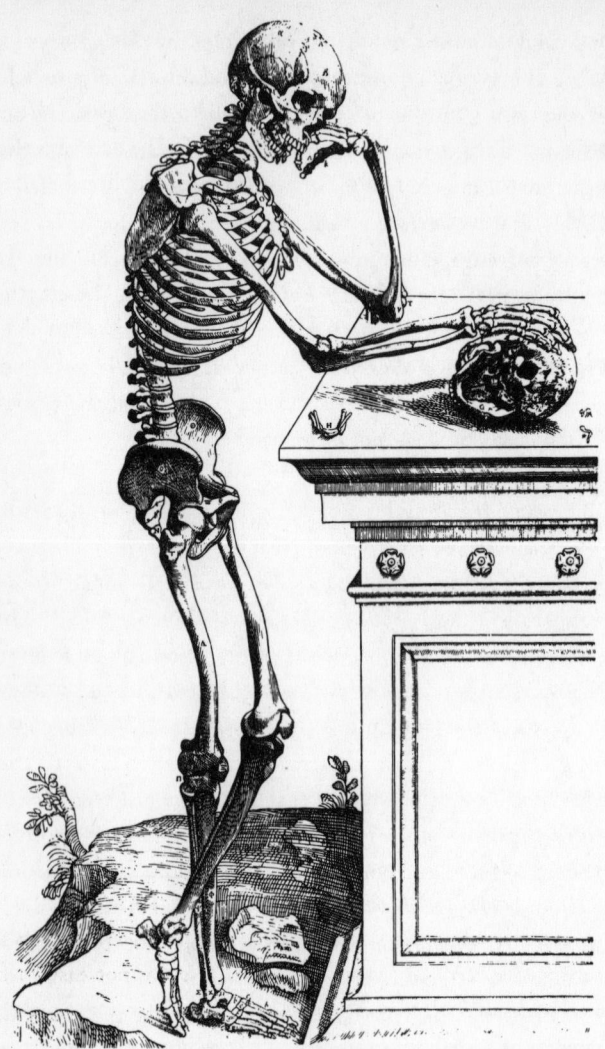

FIGURE 1. This artistically superb and anatomically exact rendering is the third skeletal drawing in Andreas Vesalius' *Fabrica*. The skeleton appears to be contemplating, or perhaps studying, the skull.

skull. These skeletons, later repeatedly plagiarized by other authors, are more than anatomical depictions; they are splendid works of art. If John Stephanus of Calcar contributed anything at all to the *Fabrica*, certainly these humanized skeletons must be from his hand. They are artistically similar to the drawings in Vesalius' earlier anatomical publication, *Tabulae anatomicae*, which Stephanus is known to have drawn.

Vesalius devotes Book 2 to a thorough description of the muscles of the human body. Thirteen muscular men display progressively the superficial and then the deeper sets of muscles. These figures in all likelihood were also drawn by John Stephanus. Like the skeleton portrayals, the "muscle men" are haunting works of art.

When Vesalius wrote that "the bad temper of sculptors and painters" made him "more miserable than the bodies he was dissecting," he probably was recalling his confrontations with artists other than Stephanus, whose talents he needed but probably failed to get in illustrating the remaining five books. Certainly there is a decided decline in the quality of the illustrations after Books 1 and 2. Not that the illustrations showing the veins and arteries in Book 3 or the nervous system in Book 4, the abdominal organs in Book 5, the heart and lungs in Book 6, and the brain in Book 7 are deficient; they just are more schematic, less distinctly human, and devoid of artistic luster.

Vesalius too often, in describing visceral organs (the liver, the kidney, the uterus), portrayed the organs of a dog or a pig rather than those of a human being. He also overlooked the presence of the pancreas, the ovaries, and the adrenal glands. These were organs rather difficult to identify, particularly in already putrefying bodies. Vesalius might have done a better job of studying the uterus, however. Admittedly, it was not easy to find dead women to dissect. Nevertheless, we know that he had the opportunity to examine the sexual organs of at least two women. For some reason, he was so anxious to dissect the hymen guarding the entrance to the vagina that he completely overlooked the uterine tubes at the other end of the genital tract. His depiction of a pregnant uterus and its fetus was medieval in its crudity.

Vesalius did very well in tracing the major arteries and veins. But his descriptions of the heart and lungs were no better than those of Galen. He was so involved in giving Greek, Latin, or Hebrew names to various muscles and tissues that he never thought of imparting his own name to any of them.

If Vesalius appeared less enthusiastic in Books 3 through 6 than he was when describing the bones and muscles in the first two books, he regained his earlier enthusiasm when he described the brain in his final book. Once more the illustrations begin to approach (but never equal) the quality of those in Books 1 and 2. Moreover, his anatomical discoveries of various parts of the brain were of supreme importance. Before Vesalius wrote Book 7, the brain's structure, as well as its functions, were almost totally unknown. With Book 7, at least some of the structural features of the brain were revealed; and henceforth the brain was no longer ignored by anatomists.

This was the *Fabrica*, a publication so scientific that it initiated medical science itself. It presented medicine with the precious gift of the scientific method with which to approach an infinite number of future medical problems. Many of the tools medical science would later employ were first developed in this revolutionary book: the complete absence of the numinous in any investigation, the straightforward unemotional prose, the exact illustration, the pitiless savagery of vivisection,[7] the need to establish priority of discovery, and the formulation of generalizations by alignment of individual observations.

The *Epitome*, a superb condensation of the *Fabrica*, was published a few weeks later. A vastly shortened volume, it was designed to be carried by medical students to the dissecting table. The *Epitome* contained several of the full-page skeletal and muscular drawings found in the *Fabrica*. It added, as resplendent ornaments, two full-page drawings: a handsome nude male (Adam) and a luscious nude woman (Eve) (see Fig. 2).

By writing the *Fabrica* and teaching directly beside his corpses on the dissection table, Vesalius was responsible for creating three Paduan successors who, within several decades after the appearance of the *Fabrica*, made major anatomical discoveries. Undeniably it was the *Fabrica* and its author who revealed the tools and the methodology that made possible these later discoveries.

The first of these luminaries was Realdo Colombo (1512–1559), successor to Vesalius at Padua. His enormous contribution, if it really was his

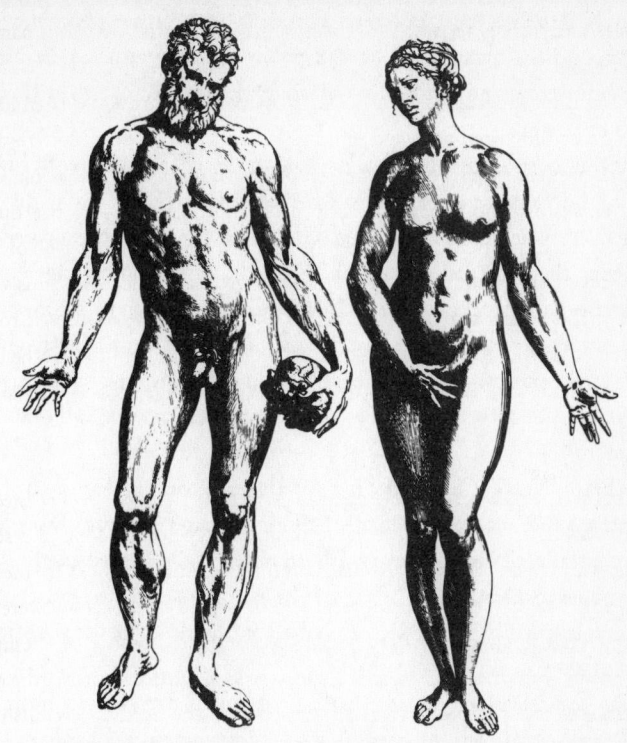

FIGURE 2. Adam and Eve as they appeared in Andreas Vesalius'
Eptome, published in 1543 conjointly with his *Fabrica*. The artist
responsible for these magnificent drawings was thought at one time
to have been Titian, but they are now attributed to Franz von Calcar.

(see Chapter 2), was the accurate description of the circulation of blood
from the right to the left ventricle of the heart via the lungs. This description, as well as detailed observation of the heart itself, first appeared
in 1559 in his posthumously published book, *De re anatomica*. We will have
more to say about Colombo in the next chapter; here, suffice it to remark
that Vesalius detested him. It was a hatred that began after Colombo accused Vesalius of not describing the tongue and eye of a human in the
Fabrica, but those of an ox.

Gabriel Fallopius (1525–1562), who succeeded Colombo to the chair of anatomy at Padua, also had been a student of Vesalius. He admired his master, and the great *Fabrica* he had published. Nevertheless, he pointed out some errors and omissions — although he was gentler than Colombo in his criticisms.

Having been taught by Vesalius how to dissect a corpse with his own hands, and to give precedence to what his own eyes saw in the dissected body over what he read in one of Galen's books, Fallopius succeeded in following these instructions so well that he observed and described quite a few anatomical processes that had escaped the attention of his master. As an example, he detected and described for the first time the ovary and the tubes of the uterus, which now bear his name. He gave the vagina, the placenta, and the clitoris the names they now bear; prior to Fallopius, they had no names.

Whereas Vesalius had *slashed* his way through what previously had been an unexplored anatomical jungle, Fallopius *threaded* his way through this now partially charted territory. He more carefully described the bones and ligaments than did Vesalius, and he even possessed the patience and meticulous curiosity to dissect out, observe, and describe the semicircular canal of the ear.

The most brilliant of all Vesalius' students, Bartolomeo Eustachius (1520–1574), was in one respect almost as unfortunate as Leonardo da Vinci. His splendid manuscript, richly adorned with copperplate engravings, finished and ready for publication in 1552, somehow or other lay completely ignored for more than one hundred fifty years in the Vatican Library. There it was discovered by the famous cardiologist Giovanni Lancisi, who published it in 1714.[8] The remarkable Eustachian discoveries were later rediscovered and published as original by anatomists of a lesser breed in the late sixteenth century and throughout the seventeenth.

Had Eustachius' book appeared in 1552 when it was first ready, it would have advanced medicine immeasurably. Indeed, its publication would have made the reputation of Eustachius almost as esteemed as that of Vesalius. Like Fallopius, Eustachius did more than just point out the errors of the *Fabrica;* he made observations that completely escaped the attention of Vesalius. His copperplate engraving of the sympathetic nervous system was an innovation of the very first rank. He also detected and provided a splendid illustration of the thoracic duct, a system that completely escaped the attention not only of Vesalius but also of William Harvey seventy-six years later. Besides the discovery of these two major systems, Eustachius correctly described the anatomy of the human kidney[9] and was the first to detect and describe the suprarenal gland and the tube bearing his name, which connects the middle ear to the oral cavity.

Of course, anatomical discoveries continued to be made after the deaths of Vesalius and his three extraordinary Paduan successors. Indeed, anatomical discoveries are still being made today. But the impetus was the publication of the *Fabrica.* So let us end this chapter with Vesalius' own words: "I could have done nothing more worthwhile than to give a new description of the whole human body, of which nobody understood the anatomy, while Galen, despite his extensive writings had offered very little on the subject, and I don't see how I could have presented my efforts to the students differently." [10]

2

William Harvey and the
Circulation of Blood

Thousands of years before the Englishman William Harvey was born, Egyptians, Greeks, and Romans not only were aware of their beating heart but attributed to it the dominant role in their spiritual and emotional activities. They believed that if humans possessed a soul, it resided in the reddish mass that pounded perpetually in one's chest. But they never troubled to find out what the beating was all about, even though they recognized that once the beating stopped, life would stop—and the soul residing in that beating heart would vanish.

Further, no Egyptian, Greek, or Roman understood what relation if any a person's blood had to this pulsating organ the size of a hand. Their essential ignorance of the functions of both the heart and the blood sprang from their failure to dissect a still-living animal. They had never directly observed the contractile and sequential movements of a living heart and the course of the blood in *both* veins and arteries. Their only knowledge of the heart and blood vessels derived from inspection of the dissected organs and tissues of human corpses. Unfortunately, the arteries of a corpse never contain blood, because when the heart ceases to beat and eject blood into the arteries, the latter contract and push all their blood into the veins.

Thus, the Egyptian, Greek, and Roman ancients, seeing no blood in the arteries of their dissected corpses, assumed that such vessels during life contained only air. Since the veins of these corpses always bulged with blood, particularly the veins entering and leaving the liver, early physicians concluded that all blood was made by this organ, which then furnished its blood, via the veins, to the other organs of the body. Recognizing that the heart must play some role in the body's economy, they postulated that it imparted a "vital spirit" to the blood entering and leaving the two chambers, or ventricles. They did not know exactly how blood entered the heart, how it traveled from the right to the left ventricle, or where it went after leaving the heart.

In the middle of the second century of our era, the Greek physician Galen made a revolutionary discovery. He observed that the right side (or right auricle) of the heart received blood from the large veins emptying into it, and that this blood was then ejected by the right ventricle into the lungs via the pulmonary artery. He further observed that the lungs drained this blood into the left side of the heart, which in turn pumped it into the aorta, the major blood vessel leaving the left ventricle.

Galen made two other cardiovascular discoveries of transcendent importance. He recognized that the heart was essentially a mass of muscles whose contraction pumped blood to and through the lungs to the left side of the heart, where again this mass of contracting muscles drove the blood into the aorta. In short, he recognized what the heart was: a pump.

His second great discovery was that, contrary to the belief of his ancient Greek and Roman forebears, arteries did not carry air; they carried blood.

Great as Galen was, he could not have detected the transit of blood from the right to the left ventricle via the lungs, or the presence of blood in arteries, merely by inspection of the organs of a dead person or animal. He had to have observed these processes in still-living people or animals. As chief physician to the gladiators of ancient Pergamum, he had the opportunity to observe these phenomena in his wounded and dying men. How often he must have noticed that when a head, arm, or leg artery was cut by sword or dagger in training or in combat, it was not air but bright, scarlet blood that spurted from the ruptured vessel. How often he must have watched the still-beating hearts of fighters who lay dying, their chests ripped open by their opponents' blades. Seeing these collapsing hearts and the adjacent lungs, how could he have failed to see the large veins pouring their purple blood into the right chamber of the heart, which then pumped this same dusky fluid directly into the collapsing lungs, which in turn poured a more brilliant red blood into the left chamber? Surely he would have observed that the left ventricle ejected its blood into the aorta, the huge artery leaving this ventricle.

Galen never disclosed that it was frequent direct observation of beating hearts and sword-savaged arteries that led to his great discoveries. He implied that it was his vivisection of animals that informed him of the cardiopulmonary and arterial events described so vividly in his writings. It was unfortunate that Galen failed to point out that his initial observations of dying *men*, not just of animals, had led to his correct understanding. Physicians for more than a thousand years believed that his descriptions depicted the cardiovascular functions of an animal, not of a person. As a consequence, these most important observations of all the hundreds of medical phenomena described by Galen in his voluminous writings were not accepted as applicable to the human heart or its blood vessels. Galen erred, moreover, in continuing to believe, as had his Greek predecessors, that the liver not only formed the body's blood, it also pumped it to the rest of the body.

So, for fourteen centuries after his death, although European physicians scrupulously accepted every one of Galen's other observations and concepts, the structure and functions of the heart, arteries, and veins continued to be matters of fantasy — precisely as they had been prior to Galen's discoveries. His observations were not lost; they remained securely, if obscurely, entrenched in his surviving writings.

They were rediscovered in the middle of the sixteenth century by Michael Servetus, a Spanish physician who even in his Parisian medical school days was recognized as possessing a knowledge of Galen's writings second to none. He also was reputed, again while still a medical student, to be extraordinarily adept in dissection of the human body.

Not only was Galen's discovery of the right-heart–lung–left-heart transit of blood (pulmonary, or lesser, circulation) accepted by Servetus, but he further confirmed its existence by pointing out that the pulmonary artery carrying blood from the right heart to the lung was too huge to carry blood to nourish only the lung. Its size indicated that it carried *all* the blood of the body to the lungs, so that the lungs could alter the blood itself. Servetus' second confirming observation was his insistence that he detected in the lung that its arteries emptied directly into its veins, which in turn emptied into the left ventricle.

Servetus was courageous enough to declare that, contrary to an age-old belief, there were no pores in the septum separating right and left ventricles. The only way blood in the right ventricle could reach the left side of the heart, he insisted, was by its transit through the pulmonary artery and lung.

Servetus described these findings in a document he wrote in 1546. Unfortunately, these precious anatomical and physiological discoveries occupied only a few paragraphs of the manuscript, which primarily was concerned with Servetus' heretical views of the nature of the Trinity and the significance of the act of baptism.

Servetus was so proud of his 1546 draft that he sent a copy to John Calvin, the Protestant pioneer. Calvin was horrified, not by the anatomical edifications of the manuscript, but by the heretical religious issues. He castigated Servetus fiercely by letter and refused to return the manuscript.

Servetus was not daunted by Calvin's stinging strictures, nor was he discouraged by Calvin's vigorous attempts to prevent publication of the manuscript. Servetus himself paid for its publication in 1553.[1]

Servetus' religious views were heretical not just to the Protestant Calvin, they also appeared heretical to the Catholic authorities. Within several months of publication of his manuscript, Servetus was arrested by French clerics. After escaping from custody during his trial, he wandered aimlessly throughout France for four months. Then, for reasons we shall never discover, he headed for Geneva, home of his most virulent enemy, John Calvin. He had not been there for more than several days when he was recognized by several monks and immediately jailed. Calvin showed him no mercy. After a trial lasting several months, he was burned at the stake on October 27, 1553, nine months after his manuscript had appeared in print.

For generations English medical historians were understandably intent on attributing to William Harvey, their countryman, total credit for discovery of the circulation of blood. They not only overlooked Galen's initial discovery of the pulmonary circulation of blood, they also insisted that Servetus' rediscovery of the same phenomenon remained unknown because *all* of his books describing this phenomenon were burned at the stake with him in 1553. But only several of these books were burned. Servetus had printed one thousand of them nine months prior to his capture. Half he had sent to a book dealer in Lyons, the other half to a dealer in Frankfurt. So certainly for many months before and probably many years after his execution, the book and its cardiovascular discoveries were not lost to the medical community.

In addition, these English protagonists, so eager to give Harvey credit for discovery of the pulmonary circulation, forgot or overlooked the fact that Servetus was in constant communication with colleagues in France, Germany, and Italy, and that it was extremely likely that he had apprised them of the pulmonary circulation during the twelve years that elapsed between his rediscovery of it and his death.

Finally, if the English Harveian enthusiasts were correct in their insistence that all Servetus' books had been destroyed, they should have been able to explain why this same book was later reprinted in both France and Germany.

It appears almost certain that Realdo Colombo, the celebrated Paduan anatomist and a contemporary of Servetus', was aware of the latter's findings long before his own observations were published posthumously in 1559,[2] six years after the printing of Servetus' book. (Even Gweneth Whitteridge, one of Harvey's most enthusiastic chroniclers, admits that Colombo was probably aware of Servetus' anatomical observations.)

Colombo did more than confirm the pulmonary circulation of blood. He made three other important observations, none of which could have been accomplished had Colombo not dissected living animals, a procedure that had not been used since Galen confirmed by animal vivisection what he had observed in dying gladiators. First, he not only revealed the presence of valves in the four vessels entering and leaving the right and left ventricles of the heart, he also discovered that these vessels permitted the flow of blood in one direction only: from the right ventricle to the lungs, back again to the left ventricle, and from there to the aorta.

Second, he correctly described the *contraction phase* of the heart ventricles (that is, the systole) and the *relaxation phase* (the diastole). Exactly when the heart contracted and when it relaxed had been a matter of total confusion for centuries prior to Colombo's delineation of this cardiac cycle.

Finally and perhaps most important, he discovered that contrary to a long-held medical opinion, the pulmonary vein leaving the lungs to empty into the left ventricle carried not a bit of air—only blood.

Colombo's 1559 book, *De re anatomica*, was distributed widely throughout Europe. There is little doubt that the Pisan botanist and anatomist Andreas Cesalpino was aware of its cardiovascular findings long before he published his own book in 1571, in which he again described the pulmonary circulation.[3] Just as Colombo failed to give Servetus credit for this discovery, Cesalpino made no mention of either Servetus or Colombo. Post-Renaissance scientists were just as ruthless in their attempts to claim priority for what they considered to be *their* discoveries as are today's Nobel laureates.

Cesalpino did make two major new observations—and one horrible mistake. His first observation was that the temporary closure of a vein in the arm or leg was followed by distension of the vein *below* the closure. It was this particular observation, later made also by William Harvey, that played such a key role in Harvey's discovery of the general circulation in the body. The critical importance of this observation was lost on Cesalpino, however. His second novel observation was that the vena cava, as it emptied into the right auricle, had a diameter wider than when it left the liver. He mistakenly concluded that this difference was proof that the vena cava carried blood *from*, not *to*, the heart.

It is virtually impossible to understand why the otherwise brilliant Italian, having observed that venous blood in the limbs of the body always traveled toward the heart, made such a mistake. We believe that this gentle botanist failed to make the greatest discovery in medicine because he could not endure the grisly task of tearing open the chests of living, suffering animals to view their still-beating hearts. Had he possessed the brazen scientific cruelty of Galen or Colombo (or Harvey a half-century later), who did resort to vivisection, those Italian medical historians who hailed Cesalpino as the real discoverer of the secret of circulation would have been correct. Because Cesalpino balked at vivisection, their championship of their countryman was and is mere chauvinistic bombast.

Long before Girolamo Fabricius, successor to Colombo at Padua, had published his book describing for the first time the valves in human veins,[4] he had observed and pointed them out to his medical students. One of his favorite students was the young Englishman William Harvey, who had just turned twenty-one. There is no question that these valves fascinated Harvey fully as much as they had Fabricius when he first detected their presence. But neither he nor Harvey (when a medical student) realized their function. This recognition finally came to Harvey several decades later; and when it did, he began to unravel the puzzle of the passage of blood in all parts of the human body.

These were the pre-Harveian pioneers and their discoveries. It is time now to learn about the life and character of William Harvey. As far as we can discover, no Englishman had ever made a significant medical discovery prior to Harvey's discovery, in the first decades of the seventeenth century, of the circulation of blood in man. He added his own observations to the earlier findings and gave birth to a concept that will endure forever.

Unfortunately, Harvey's personal belongings were destroyed—first in 1642 by Oliver Cromwell's soldiers, and again in 1666 by the huge London fire that burned the library of the Royal College of Physicians (where almost all of Harvey's personal and scientific papers and books were kept). What remains is several of his letters, and some scattered and usually brief accounts of a few of his activities and remarks, as remembered by three of his contemporaries: Robert Boyle, the founder of modern chemistry; John Aubrey, a not too reliable, gossipy sort of historian; and Sir George Ent, a devoted medical disciple of Harvey's. In addition to Harvey's masterpiece, *De motu cordis*, the two other books he published are extant. Miraculously saved from the 1666 fire are notes prepared for his 1616 Lumley anatomical lectures to the physicians of the Royal College, now securely housed in the

British Museum. It is from these surviving artifacts and a few other data that William Harvey and his activities can be described.

Harvey was born in 1578 at Folkestone, a small and very ancient town several miles from Dover. The eldest of seven brothers, he showed himself early on to be a brilliant youngster. He was awarded a scholarship to Caius College (Cambridge), where he received his undergraduate degree. Although the college was given two hanged criminals each year for dissection, Harvey did not remain there for medical training. He traveled to Padua, where Vesalius and then Colombo had successively held the chair of anatomy. Harvey was well aware of their discoveries. He became Fabricius' assistant in 1600, and Fabricius was one of the four professors who signed Harvey's diploma. Harvey himself wrote "1578" as his birth date on the diploma, the only source for his year of birth.

At age twenty-four he returned to London. He was quite short, had very dark brown eyes, jet-black hair, and a disposition that was not too pleasing. John Aubrey described him as choleric and ever ready to reach for the dagger that he always carried. Even the medical historian who admired him most, Geoffrey Keynes, described him as "aloof."

He married quite well, in that he took as his bride Elizabeth Browne, whose father was an attending physician to Queen Elizabeth. With such a celebrated father-in-law, Harvey was quickly accepted as a Fellow of the Royal College of Physicians. He soon became the attending physician at Saint Bartholomew's Hospital and after Queen Elizabeth's death was one of the royal physicians attending James I. When James died in 1625 (Harvey participated in his autopsy), Harvey became one of the physicians attending Charles I.

He might well have attained these positions even if he had not married Dr. Browne's daughter. From the beginning of his career he was deeply respected for his scientific knowledge, as evidenced by his annual invitation, beginning in 1616, to give the Royal College's Lumley lectures.

Almost nothing is known about his wife, Elizabeth, except that she kept and dearly loved a parrot that Harvey describes in great detail in his embryology book. When the parrot died suddenly, Harvey dissected the bird. To his surprise, he discovered that the parrot, which he always had believed to be a male bird (because she sang and talked), had died from a decaying egg in her oviduct. This finding prompted Harvey to believe that she had died for lack of love; he quoted six lines of Virgil that commented on spring and its awakening of the Venus in everyone.

A portrait of Mrs. Harvey and her parrot was destroyed by fire in 1907; it would have been interesting to gaze at this probably lovely mate of Harvey's. It is likely that hers was not a rapturously happy marriage. There were no children, only a parrot and a husband absent from her for years and obsessed with the continuous dissection of more than a hundred different species of animals ranging from fleas to deer and including snakes, snails, geese, turtles, fishes, and rats. Then too it might not have been blissful to live with a man who frequently remarked to John Aubrey that Europeans "know not how to order or govern" their women, and that the Turks were the only people who "used them wisely." One does not get the sense that Harvey was an ardent feminist!

Harvey could not have been a totally likable person. He, like the vivisectionist Claude Bernard two centuries later, had to be pitiless. Otherwise how could he have withstood the wails, shrieks, groans, and moans of the unanesthetized dogs and other animals he ruthlessly vivisected? Perhaps Harvey's wife, like the wife and daughter of Bernard, detested him because of this sort of cruelty.

It is of interest too that although Harvey's colleagues at the Royal College greatly admired his scientific achievements and even during his lifetime employed the adjectives "divine" and "immortal" in speaking of him, they did not offer him the presidency of the Royal College until its members were certain that he was too old (age seventy-three) to accept their offer.

Just how skilled a physician Harvey was is unclear. Aubrey wrote that although he was admired as a scientist, Harvey was not esteemed as a therapist. He certainly had not freed himself from some medieval medical beliefs. Thus he reported that a breast tumor had vanished after he had stroked it with the cold hand of a corpse. But he preceded present-day medical thinking when he eradicated another tumor *by depriving it of its blood supply.*

Harvey also believed in witches; at the request of King Charles I, he gladly agreed to examine a suspected witch. Like his contemporaries, he searched the woman's body for one of two corporeal blemishes that witches were supposed to exhibit: segments of calloused body skin that were insensitive to pain, or teats at sites other than the breasts or chest. Harvey thought he had discovered such a teat adjacent to what he described as "her secrets" (the witch's genitals), but on closer examination the suspected teat proved to be a harmless withered hemorrhoidal skin flap.

For better or for worse, Harvey had the personality of a scientist. He was profoundly absorbed in plucking from nature's vast collection as many facts as he could possibly obtain. He was not interested in what his friends (or even his king) were doing with their lives. For example, in 1635, while Charles I was at Edgehill, battling for his kingdom and his life, Harvey sat under a hedge calmly reading a book until the close falling of bullets forced him to move farther back.

Toward the end of his life he was talking with John Aubrey about his past. It was not the marvel of his life with Elizabeth or his sorrow at her death that persisted in his memory, but the loss in 1642 of a manuscript dealing with insects that he had almost completed writing. Aubrey reported that Harvey told him that this loss "was the greatest crucifying" he had endured in his entire life. It was the lament of a true scientist, whose genuine pleasure in life was a continuous attempt to discover and understand as many of nature's entities and processes as possible. Harvey resorted chiefly to dissection and vivisection of every species of animal he could get his hands on, whether a shrimp, a toad, or the 152-year-old Thomas Parr.

He spent the last seven of his seventy-nine years living at the home of Eliab, his only surviving brother, who was very wealthy. Eliab maintained his own male servant and also, according to John Aubrey, "kept a pretty, young wench to wayte [sic] on him which I guess he made use of for warmth-sake, as King David did. . . ."

Dr. George Ent, the young and devoted admirer of Harvey, on visiting the retired physician in 1649 happened to notice that Harvey possessed a large but disorderly collection of embryological studies. Ent immediately recognized the singular importance of these empirical and experimental observations, and he at length succeeded in getting Harvey to agree to Ent's editing and publishing a book that would describe Harvey's multifarious embryological studies. The volume was published in 1651.[5] In this book too, Harvey presented a totally new concept: that all life originated from and first developed in an egg or an ovum. Unlike the circulation of blood, this embryological concept was not confirmed until 1827, when Carl Baer discovered the ovum in the human ovary.

Harvey died of a stroke in 1657. He was buried in the vault below a chapel that Eliab had erected as an addition to the Hempstead Church in Essex. With the passage of years, the windows of the vault were broken, exposing Harvey's lead-encased body to wind-driven rain as well as to rocks hurled by youngsters. Such maltreatment eventually cracked Harvey's lead coffin. Upon discovering this situation, the Fellows of the Royal College of Physicians sought to remove the damaged coffin from the vault and inter it at Westminster Abbey. They were not able to accomplish this transfer, so in solemn procession they carried the coffin from the vault to the chapel directly above it. There they deposited it in an elaborate marble sarcophagus, in which William Harvey will lie forever.

Harvey's true monument was his *De motu cordis*. Within the span of just seventeen years in the first third of the seventeenth century, the three greatest books of the English language were published: King James's authorized version of the Bible (1611); the Folio Edition of Shakespeare's plays (1623); and the English translation of William Harvey's *Exercitatio anatomica de motu cordis et sanguinis in animalibus* (1628), which for centuries afterward was universally known as *De motu cordis*. And what the authorized version of the Bible has been to the Church of England and the Shakespeare Folio to English literature, *De motu cordis* has been to medicine everywhere.

Before this badly printed (126 errors in the first edition), seventy-two-page, seventeen-chapter book appeared, no significant medical book had ever been published by an English scholar. Probably two hundred copies were printed, of which (according to Geoffrey Keynes) only fifty-three have survived. Even some of these lack the first page, on which Harvey obsequiously paid his respects to King Charles I. We believe that the excision was performed on those of Harvey's books that came into the hands of ardent Scotch Presbyterians, who could not abide even a printed dedication to the Catholic-leaning Charles.

Exactly when Harvey decided to publish *De motu cordis* is ambiguous, but we do know that by deliberate design he preceded its publication with twelve years of lecturing to his colleagues at the Royal College of Physicians about the heart, arteries, and veins. In the course of these lectures he presented vivisections in which the timid but fascinated Fellows could see blood gushing from the right ventricle of a living, shrieking pig, into its lungs, then into the left ventricle, to be ejected into the aorta and its arterial branches.

In his dedication of De motu cordis, Harvey cited these repeated exposures of Royal College physicians to his lectures and experiments to no less a dignitary than Dr. Argent, the president of the Royal College:

> I have already and repeatedly presented to you, my learned friends, my new views of the motion and function of the heart, in my anatomical lectures; but having now for nine years and more confirmed these views by multiple demonstrations in your presence, illustrated them by arguments, and freed them from the objections of the most learned and skilful anatomists, I at length yield to the requests, I might say entreaties of many, and here present them for general consideration in this treatise.

Harvey was well aware that it might be perilous for an English physician to contradict the centuries-old doctrines of Galen. At the very least, such a medical heresy would lead to expulsion from the Royal College. So he very cautiously, very patiently, and very masterfully succeeded in convincing every single member of the college of the ineluctable correctness of all his concepts. He thus was assured that come what might from foreign critics of his published views, the best medical minds in England—those possessed by the physicians of the Royal College—would loyally defend him and his revolutionary concepts.

He took further precautions in writing his monograph. He never once *directly* ridiculed a single view or concept of Galen. Quite aware that not only Galen but also Servetus, Colombo, and Cesalpino had described the pulmonary or lesser circulation, Harvey gave only Galen some credit for this discovery. Similarly, although he was cognizant of Colombo's discovery that arteries contained no air but only blood, he again attributed this discovery to Galen, his ancient predecessor and fellow vivisectionist. It is only on close perusal of De motu cordis and reflection on its contents that one realizes that despite Harvey's treacly praise of Galen, he relentlessly presented his own observations, ranging from the dying heart of a snake to the exposed but beating heart of Viscount Hugh Montgomery. In so doing, he succeeded in totally destroying most of Galen's concepts of the heart's structure and functions.

Harvey, besides his years of expounding and proving the validity of his own concepts to his college associates and always being very careful to praise Galen's greatness even as he destroyed his concepts, also took exquisite pains to withhold in *De motu cordis* his own original and magnificent discovery, until he set a proper stage for its appearance by writing the book's first seven chapters. He described in those chapters the anatomy and workings of the auricles, ventricles, arteries, veins, and valves of the heart. Let us glance at these chapters before proceeding to the eighth, in which he announced the discovery that made medicine begin to move as a science.

In the seven introductory chapters Harvey very smoothly (if one were brutally frank, one could substitute "cunningly" for "smoothly") portrayed the anatomy of the auricles, ventricles, and blood vessels of the heart. He also described the valves of blood vessels entering and leaving the heart's chambers. He then wrote of the semilunar valves of the pulmonary artery and pointed out that the manner of their opening and closing indicated that the pulmonary artery must carry blood *to* the lungs *from* the right ventricle. He did not mention that Colombo, of whose earlier observations of the heart he was well aware, had described the structure and function of these semilunar valves sixty-nine years earlier. Perhaps Harvey felt justified in plagiarizing Colombo's findings because he assuredly knew that Colombo had failed to give credit to Servetus for his original description of the same vascular structure. Harvey in these first seven chapters also emphasized that the heart's only function was to pump blood and he clearly differentiated the contractions of the auricles from those of the ventricles, noting that the auricles contracted *before* the ventricles. This last observation was truly novel. Prior to Harvey's studies, no one could determine whether or not the auricles contracted before the ventricles because the hearts of most vivisected animals beat so rapidly that the sequence of contractions could not be discerned.

Harvey solved this difficulty in two ways. First, he dissected and observed the far more slowly beating hearts of cold-blooded animals, such as fish. Second, Harvey waited patiently until his vivisected warm-blooded animals began to die, at which time their heart's contractions became slower and slower. It was in such dying animals that Harvey observed that the auricle contracted first, ejecting its blood into its contiguous ventricle, after which the ventricle contracted.

Having reported the heart's anatomy and function, as well as the pulsation of arteries, Harvey described in his sixth and seventh chapters the dynamics of the pulmonary or lesser circulation; that is, the transit of blood from the right heart via the lungs to the left heart. So masterly was his prose and so closely did he weave his demonstrations of cardiac anatomy and dynamics in the first five chapters—and so complete was his failure to refer to the identical observations of Servetus, Colombo, and Cesalpino—that his account of the pulmonary circulation in chapters 6 and 7 dazzled the reader as Harvey's own totally triumphant, original discovery. So artfully written was his reference to Galen's discovery of the same lesser circulation that Galen appeared to be confirming Harvey's findings, not preceding them by more than fourteen hundred years. (His literary cunning did not mislead the distinguished anatomist William Hunter, however. Hunter pointed out in 1783 that it was not Harvey but Colombo and Cesalpino who had first discovered the pulmonary circulation.)

In chapter 8 Harvey warned that his next words would be "of so novel and unheard-of character, that I not only fear injury to myself from the envy of a few, but I tremble lest I have mankind at large for my enemies." He then announced:

> *I began to think whether there might be a motion, as it were, in a circle.* Now this I afterwards found to be true; and I finally saw that the blood, forced by action of the left ventricle into the arteries, was distributed to the body at large, . . . *and it then passed through the veins and along the vena cava, and so round to the left ventricle* in the manner already indicated. Which motion we may be allowed to call *circular.*

Harvey, after presenting this glittering concept as a flash of intuition, proceeded in fascinating fashion in the subsequent nine chapters to settle for all time its puissant validity. Never before, and very rarely since, has a scientist presented his experimental results in language so lucid and yet so elegant.

Harvey's first, brilliant experiment leading to the concept of *circulation* was to measure the blood in the left ventricle of a dog's heart. Multiplying this approximate quantity by the number of heartbeats per minute, he calculated that this left ventricle would eject three pounds of blood in just half an hour, a quantity almost equal to the total blood volume of the animal. Harvey then, almost rhetorically and certainly decisively, asked whence all the blood leaving the left ventricle could be coming. It could not be from the food and liquids ingested. How could the aorta and its arteries accept such a huge amount of blood without ridding itself quickly of most of the blood it received? The only logical answer was that the blood the heart ejected into the aorta and arteries returned via the veins to the heart, thus completing Harvey's precious "*circle.*"

Harvey followed these measurements and calculations with direct observations of what happened to the beating heart of a living snake when he temporarily occluded the single vein leading to it. He found that the heart paled, shrank, and stopped ejecting blood into its aorta. When the occlusion was removed, the heart immediately resumed its purplish-red color and again pumped blood into the aorta. When the aorta in turn was occluded, its segment proximal to the occlusion, as well as the heart itself, swelled with blood obstructed by the aortic occlusion. These observations again demonstrated that the heart ejected blood into the arterial system only after receiving this blood from the venous system.

Harvey's subsequent investigations of the flow of blood in peripheral veins and arteries added further substance to his concept of the circulation of blood. He pointed out that when a vein was ligated, the segment below the ligature always swelled; the segment above the ligature always collapsed. Even more telling, when he ligated an artery, the veins connected to this artery always collapsed, only to open and fill with blood as soon as the ligature was removed (see Fig. 3).

It was in his chapter 13 that Harvey described the simple experiments that many years later he told John Boyle, England's most celebrated chemist, gave him the idea that blood flows in a continuous circle from arteries to veins and back again.

Before he proceeded in this chapter to describe the critical experiments, he pointed out that the valves of all the body's veins were so constructed that they allowed the flow of blood in one direction only. He proved this thesis by showing that he could pass a probe in only one direction in a vein, namely the direction toward which the vein valves opened.

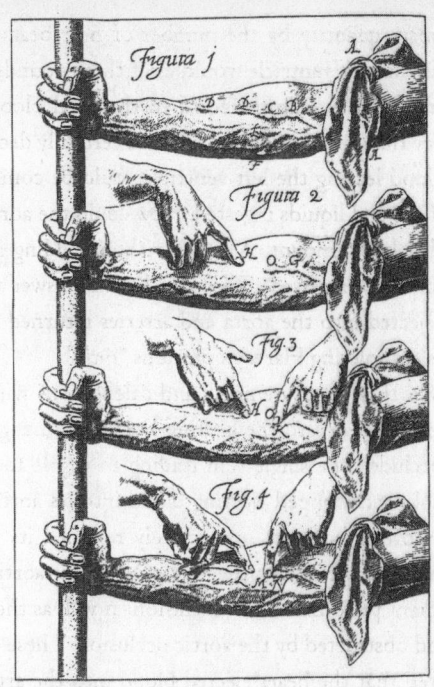

FIGURE 3. This drawing of an arm whose
veins and valves are distended by a tourniquet is
the only illustration in William Harvey's book
De motu cordis. His observations of the swelling of
a vein below an obstruction and its collapse
above first led him to suspect that all the blood
in veins was flowing to the heart.

But in which direction did these valves permit the blood to flow? Harvey's simple but crucial experiments provided the answer.

He first applied a ligature to a man's upper arm, tightly enough to obliterate its pulse. The arm lost its color and warmth and became painful. More important, Harvey observed that the arm veins collapsed. When the ligature was loosened a bit to allow some arterial blood to flow, the arm and hand below the ligature became warm and regained their previous color. The arm veins in turn became distended with blood whose escape was still prevented by the partially loosened ligature.

Harvey believed that this experiment clearly showed that arterial blood entered and nourished the arm and later flowed into the veins. But in what direction did the blood flow in the arm veins? Harvey found the answer to this critical question by applying a tourniquet lightly on the upper arm of a human volunteer. He waited until the veins of the arm swelled, revealing the location of its valves. With his left index finger he occluded a vein at the site of one of its valves. With his right index finger he pressed upward all the blood in the vein segment above the occluded valve, up to and slightly beyond the next valve above the occluded lower valve. Removing his right index finger, he noted that the vein segment between the two valves remained collapsed. Thus the upper valve did not permit blood to flow back to the collapsed vein segment. When, however, he removed his left finger from the lower valve, the collapsed vein segment above it quickly filled. Harvey now knew that venous blood always flowed back to the heart.

This simple experiment confirmed what Harvey had discovered earlier in his numerous vivisections. The valves of all veins—in the limbs, the abdomen, the chest, and even the head—permitted flow in only one direction, *toward* the heart. When this fact was joined with the observation that arterial blood also flowed in only one direction, *away* from the heart, there could be only one dynamic explanation: the blood flowed in a circle.

Harvey's chapter 14 contained just two sentences, the second of which announced his final conclusion:

Since all things, both argument and ocular demonstration, show that the blood passes through the lungs and heart by the action of the [auricles and] ventricles, and is sent for distribution to all parts of the body, where it makes its way into the veins and pores of the flesh, and then flows by the veins from the circumference on every side to the center, from the lesser to the greater veins, and is by them finally discharged into the vena cava and right auricle of the heart, and this in such a quantity or in such a flux and reflux thither by the arteries, hither by the veins, as cannot possibly be supplied by the ingesta, and in much greater than can be required for mere purposes of nutrition; it is absolutely necessary to conclude that the blood is in a state of ceaseless motion; that this is the act or function which the heart performs by means of its pulse; and that is the sole and only end of the motion and contraction of the heart.

This summarizing sentence is the most significant medical declaration ever published. Vesalius gave medicine a magnificent representation of the body; but it portrayed a body functionally transmogrified by death into a motionless mass of muscle and bone enclosing a heterogeneous collection of organs and tissues. Their multifarious functions were to remain totally mysterious for another eighty-five years, until Harvey's immortal sentence gave life and motion to two of the body's most important components, its heart and its blood.

We have already mentioned that Harvey took pains to ensure that all his colleagues at the Royal College were apprised of his views concerning not only the lesser but also the general circulation. So he received no stinging criticism from his English contemporaries, although those of his own generation did not actively defend him from the European contemporaries who bitterly maligned his book.

European critics did not attack his views on the lesser circulation; they knew that Galen, Servetus, Colombo, and Cesalpino had already demonstrated the passage of blood from the right to the left heart via the lungs. What they malevolently assailed was Harvey's description of the general circulation—that *all* the blood flowed from the arteries of the entire body to the veins, and back again via the heart to the arteries. They still believed that the liver was ejecting blood for circulation throughout the body. (It is only fair to point out that Harvey himself was not totally clear about the liver and its handling of blood and chyle, the milky fluid derived from foods digested in the intestines. Chyle leaves the intestines via the lymphatic vessels, which were first observed and described in 1627 by Caspare Aselli.) In 1616, Harvey believed as did his contemporaries that the liver supplied blood *to* the intestines and received chyle *from* the intestines, the two fluids flowing in opposite directions in the portal vein. Sometime after 1620, but before 1628, Harvey changed his mind. He then insisted that the portal vein carried blood *from* the intestines and *to* the liver. Still believing that chyle also traveled in the portal vein to the liver, he refused to accept Aselli's discovery of the intestinal lymphatic vessels and their transport of chyle to the thoracic duct.

It is more than likely that Harvey had concentrated so intensely on demonstrating the circular movement of blood from the veins to the arteries that he forgot to mention in his book the difference in color of the venous and the arterial blood. His anatomist predecessors assuredly had recognized this color difference. Even his immortal contemporary Shakespeare was aware of the dusky red color of venous blood; in *Julius Caesar* he has Brutus whisper to Portia, "You are as dear to me as the *ruddy* drops that visit my sad heart."

Or perhaps the reason for Harvey's failure to mention the difference in color of venous and arterial blood was his total ignorance of the lung's role in aerating the blood passing through it. Forty-one years later Richard Lower would demonstrate that venous blood passing through the lungs changed its dark blue color to a bright scarlet because of exposure to air in its pulmonary passage.[6] He later proved this fact very simply by collecting venous blood in an open flask and shaking it; the dusky violet color immediately changed to a brilliant red.

Harvey also had to assume that the body's arteries emptied into the veins. He was unable to observe such connections because the microscope had not yet been invented. The Italian anatomist Marcello Malpighi, however, in 1661 did have a microscope; with it he detected the tiny capillaries through which blood in the arteries flowed to reach the veins.[7] With this discovery Harvey's circle had been completed.

3

Antony Leeuwenhoek and Bacteria

                                           Regnier de Graaf lived only thirty-
two years, but during that brief period this Dutch physician and anatomist
not only succeeded in discovering the egg-bearing sites of the ovary but
was indirectly responsible for bringing the microbe to the attention of the
medical world. In 1673, just a few months before he died, he wrote a letter to
Henry Oldenburg, the secretary of the Royal Society of London, inform-
ing him that a fellow Dutchman had constructed a marvelous microscope
with which he was able to see wondrously small objects. It is doubtful
that de Graaf also informed Oldenburg that this countryman, Antony van
Leeuwenhoek, was not a professor or a physician but an unlearned shop-
keeper selling dry goods, who knew no languages except his native Dutch.

    Because of de Graaf's fame and reputation, Oldenburg invited Leeuwen-
hoek to submit a letter reporting some of his microscopic findings for
possible publication in the society's *Philosophical Transactions*.

Leeuwenhoek undoubtedly was flattered by Oldenburg's invitation. Yet in submitting his first paper in 1673, he wrote that previously he had not tried to publish any of his findings because he was unsure of his ability to express himself effectively—and also because he did not like to be contradicted. Fortunately the first report of this eccentric Dutch haberdasher contained little to criticize; he described the appearance of a common mold, as well as the eye, sting, and mouth of a bee, as seen through his microscope. Actually, these first observations of Leeuwenhoek were not as dramatic as those published earlier, in 1664, by Robert Hooke, a Fellow of the Royal Society.[1]

Before we continue our account of the scientific achievements of the amazing Antony Leeuwenhoek, let us relate a few details of his life. He lived to be ninety-one years of age, having been born in 1632 and died in 1723 (see Fig. 4). Such longevity, while not unique, was no mean feat for a person living then or even now. He married his first wife, Barbara, when he was twenty-two; she died twelve years later and he married again a few years afterward. Of his five children by his first wife, only Maria survived. After his second wife died, Maria (who never married) lived with her father and cared for him for the rest of his life.

Although not well educated, Leeuwenhoek was respected as a man of integrity by the citizenry of Delft. He was especially well known to the members of the council that governed Delft. In 1676 they appointed him trustee of the bankrupt estate of the widow of the still-to-be-recognized painter Jan Vermeer.

Leeuwenhoek probably lived as pleasant a life as any of his fellow burghers. He drank scalding hot coffee at breakfast and tea in the late afternoon. He had no fear of cholesterol-rich foods, nor did he confine himself to unsaturated fats. And he had what so many of us lack today— unconditional love and affection. Maria, his daughter, adored him. In addition, he enjoyed the loyalty of his long-haired dog, a talking parrot, and his gentle horse. His work as a draper, hardly consuming, left him well over 120,000 hours to expend during his sixty-one years of making microscopes. He would peer through them at such disparate objects as the lens of a whale, his own sperm, and the manure of his horse. In his shop were no telephones, no incessantly clicking computerized cash registers, and no government or insurance forms of any kind to distract him as he ground

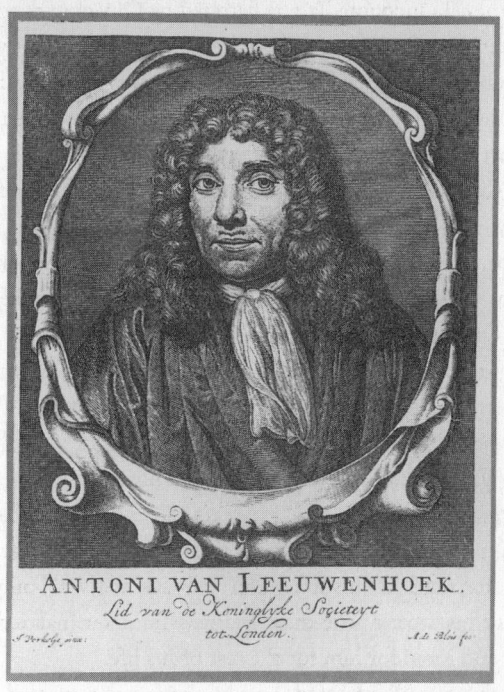

ANTONI VAN LEEUWENHOEK.
*Lid van de Koninglycke Societeyt
tot Londen.*

FIGURE 4. Engraving of Antony Leeuwenhoek as it
appeared in his six-volume series of books, *Ontledingen
en Ontdekkwegen,* 1693.

hundreds of convex lenses and wrote long letters for publication in the
Philosophical Transactions of the Royal Society.

Perhaps Leeuwenhoek was not a very enterprising draper. We do not
know or care how many bolts of cloth or how many hats he sold. These
were not what Maria tabulated on the white marble monument that marks
his grave in the yard of the Old Church of Delft. Rather, she had engraved,
on a plaque attached to the tall obelisk, that her father astonished the
world by employing a microscope to discover new and strikingly important secrets of nature. This simple, uneducated daughter thereby forecast
what we recognize today: her father first recognized a world of creatures
who had been and still are responsible for the illnesses and deaths of un-
told millions of men and women.

For fifty years Leeuwenhoek continued to send his now-famous scientific letters to the Royal Society. Written in Dutch, they were translated into English or Latin for publication in the *Philosophical Transactions*. Even as he lay dying at age ninety-one, he begged his physician to translate into Latin several letters written in Dutch, prior to their transmission to the Royal Society.

Several years before his death, Leeuwenhoek fashioned a lovely wooden cabinet with a number of shelves to hold twenty-six of his different microscopes, many of which bore lenses mounted in silver. Each of these microscopes had objects permanently affixed to it for easy viewing: a segment of a hog's tongue, the eye of a flea, and a crystallized section of the vitreous humor of a whale's eye. Maria, dutifully following her father's wishes, dispatched this precious cabinet to London within weeks of his death. It was housed at the Royal Society for over a century before it mysteriously disappeared. Besides the microscopes given to the society, Leeuwenhoek at his death had accumulated 247 others and 172 lenses mounted in gold, silver, and brass. Maria put these microscopes and lenses up for auction in 1745; they brought in 61 pounds.

Leeuwenhoek did not live the obscure, poverty-stricken life endured by Vermeer, his fellow townsman. He knew his discoveries were monumental and that sooner or later their landmark significance would be recognized. Even in his lifetime, an emperor and Queen Mary of England visited his quaint draper's shop. Other royal and noble personages too visited him to view the invisible world he had unveiled. As a part-time scientist, he almost certainly lived a far gentler, more tranquil and spiritually satisfying life than the majority of Nobel laureates today.

But enough about the life of this draper-researcher who never forgot to throw bread crumbs on the snow for the hungry sparrows that flocked about his house. Let us now describe his famous Letter 18, which gave this humble man the precious gift of immortality.

This letter—17½ folio pages bearing Leeuwenhoek's handwritten Dutch—was received by Henry Oldenburg of the Royal Society in October 1676. He proceeded to translate it into English, after condensing it to half.[2] The translated, condensed letter appeared in the society's March 1677 *Philosophical Transactions*.

Letter 18 begins simply enough: "In the year 1675, about half-way through September . . . I discovered little creatures in rain which had stood but a few days in a new tub that was painted blue within." Leeuwenhoek decided to investigate this phenomenon further because he saw that "these little animals to my eye were more than ten thousand times smaller than . . . the water-flea or water-louse, which you can see alive and moving in water with the bare eye."

He continued his microscopic investigation not only of rainwater, but also of water from his well and seawater. All these different specimens had been left exposed to the air prior to his microscopic scrutiny. He was particularly fascinated by the "little animals" he saw that possessed tiny "legs" or "tails" which allowed them to scurry here, there, and everywhere in the tiny drop of water that was their world. He even pitied a particular protozoan that became entangled in microscopic debris and was not able to extricate itself.

The major portion of Letter 18 is composed of Leeuwenhoek's diary entries between September 1675 and September 1676, describing his various experiments. It is not until he examined water that had been infused with ground pepper that he described microscopic "animals" that were without question bacteria. Their immobility, or sluggish motion at best, puzzled Leeuwenhoek, who was not always sure that they were living creatures. There was no question that he preferred those of his little animals that had heads and tails and moved swiftly. At no time in this particular letter did he even suspect that his little animals had "cousins" that have been among man's deadliest enemies.

It may be difficult for us today, accustomed since childhood to be mindful of all our microscopic friends (certain yeasts, molds, and some bacteria) and enemies (the tetanus and diphtheria bacilli, not to forget the spirochete of syphilis), to understand how surprising—even incredible—Letter 18 was for the eminently pragmatic minds of the Fellows of the Royal Society. "Here is this letter from an unlearned Dutch draper whom we really don't know, in which he claims to have detected thousands of animals in a tiny drop of rain water. He must send us verification of these findings by others whom we can trust!" Thinking along these lines, the members requested that Leeuwenhoek invite some of his more illustrious fellow townsmen to his home and demonstrate the existence of his little animals so that they could authenticate his microscopic findings to the society.

Leeuwenhoek did exactly that, inviting several of Delft's most respected citizens (including the minister of his church) to his home. Not only did the committee uphold Leeuwenhoek's observations, but Robert Hooke, the society's own microscopist, in 1678 verified the findings.

Two years after Hooke's confirmation of the epochal observations described in this famous Letter 18, Leeuwenhoek was invited to become a Fellow of the Royal Society. Neither before this invitation nor to the present day has this most prestigious of all scientific societies ever invited a haberdasher and part-time janitor to enter its membership ranks. How inexpressibly proud Leeuwenhoek must have been on receiving such recognition! He showed his gratitude by submitting more papers during his fifty years of membership than any other Fellow in the three hundred years and more of the society's existence.

Many of Leeuwenhoek's papers were almost as important as his Letter 18. For example, in his Letter 39, submitted to the society in 1683, he described examining under his microscope his own spittle and scrapings from plaque adhering to his front teeth. Although he discerned no little animals in his spittle, the scrapings from his plaque were alive with thousands of them. He later noted that when he reexamined the scrapings, he was no longer able to detect any little animals.

"What happened to the little animals that I earlier saw in the scrapings?" he asked himself over and over. Then one morning he believed he knew the answer. Several days after his initial findings he had taken up the habit of drinking scalding coffee every morning. "The heat of that coffee probably killed my little animals," he said to himself. If this were the reason for his failure later to find microscopic creatures in the scrapings from his front teeth, then the plaque adhering to the teeth at the back of his mouth, not directly exposed to the scalding coffee, might still harbor little animals. How excited Leeuwenhoek became when, on examining the scrapings from one of his rear teeth, he found myriad "animalcules" therein.

There is little question that Leeuwenhoek came within a few cerebral neurons of discovering that his little animals did more than just flock to "corrupted" flesh and bone, that they were responsible for the corruption in the first place. How near he was to this germ concept of disease is revealed by his report of animalcules in the scrapings from his coated tongue when he was ill and feverish. And again, when extracting one of his rotten teeth and examining with his microscope the pultaceous decay of its roots, he recognized once more his microscopic denizens—multiplied to the hundreds of thousands.

Leeuwenhoek in his fifty years of association with the Royal Society achieved far more than his discovery of the microscopic world of living creatures. He examined not only his own feces but also those of cows, horses, and pigeons. Only the dung of horses and cows harbored none of his little animals. He studied his own blood and was surprised to see that it consisted in great part of what we know as red blood cells; he noted that under his microscope these cells lost their scarlet color.

It was the microscopic examination of his semen that surprised him. It too swarmed with little animals. But in contrast to what he had seen in rain, seawater, or well water, the animalcules of his semen were all alike. All of the thousands at which he peered had identical tails, and bodies consisting essentially of only a head; and all were moving hither and yon in the drop of his seminal fluid. It took the university-based savants quite a few decades to accept Leeuwenhoek's discovery of the existence of these restless sperm creatures. Of course, none of the disbelievers ever took the trouble to examine their own semen under a microscope.

The reader may wonder why other scientists, who had had microscopes at their disposal for a full half-century, failed to discern the existence of creatures invisible to the human eye. Certainly some of their microscopes were more sophisticated than the simple biconvex lens system fabricated by Leeuwenhoek. The answer is simple enough: they would only examine an object, minute as it might be, that they could see unaided—whether that object was the egg of a silkworm or the eye of a louse. They had not divined as Leeuwenhoek had that objects of some kind might exist in liquids such as water, blood, and semen that were invisible to the eye alone.

We can see now that this sublimely simple Dutch draper and part-time janitor was rightly designated the founder of bacteriology and proto-zoology by his biographer, Clifford Dobell, and also by William Bullock, author of the finest book available on the history of bacteriology.[3] But on his death in 1723, Leeuwenhoek was promptly forgotten not only by the Royal Society and the rest of the learned world, but even by his own countrymen, his own townsmen. Only the obelisk over his grave in Delft, erected by his devoted daughter in 1745, reminds us that this truly great man, in his ninety-one incredibly fertile years, discovered a hitherto unknown universe of living creatures.

Thirty-nine years after Leeuwenhoek's death an Austrian, Marc von Plenciz (1705–1781), declared flatly that contagious diseases were caused by the Dutchman's small animalcules. This article of Plenciz's, or possibly Leeuwenhoek's own publications in the *Philosophical Transactions of the Royal Society*, did not escape the attention of Agostino Bassi (1773–1836) of Lodi, Italy. In a seminal study, Bassi demonstrated experimentally in 1835 that silkworm disease was caused by bacteria. By inference he postulated that other diseases also might be caused by bacteria. At last, after 112 years, some of Leeuwenhoek's little animals were identified as the cause of infection.

These findings were appreciated by Friedrich Henle (1809–1885), Europe's foremost anatomist of the time. There is little question that Henle impressed on his most brilliant student, Robert Koch, the earthshaking implications of Bassi's work. Koch soon took up the torch first ignited by Leeuwenhoek in 1676. And when Koch had made his own landmark discoveries, Antony van Leeuwenhoek's ghost could lie at peace — because Koch's work ensured that Leeuwenhoek's achievements would be remembered forever.

Louis Pasteur, if nothing else, was a true Frenchman: quick-tempered, egotistical, obsessively intense, and so patriotic that after the Franco-Prussian War in 1870, he swore he would write at the beginning of all his scientific papers, "Hatred to the Prussians." Although given to hasty decisions and flights of fancy, he could be fully as methodical and as patient as his hated Prussians were reputed to be. And he was extraordinarily adept at profiting from the gifts of serendipity.

Pasteur was born in 1822 in the small village of Dole, the son of a tanner. In elementary school, and later in secondary school, he showed no aptitude whatsoever for the physical sciences. But he did possess a fine talent for drawing. Despite this truly exquisite ability, his goal was to matriculate someday at the Sorbonne and learn to be a chemist. He enrolled in a preparatory school for later entrance into the Sorbonne, but during his first few months became so homesick that he returned to Dole. There he savored again that which he had missed most, the acrid smells of his father's tanning works.

After just several months, he returned to the same preparatory school, where his grades subsequently were at least tolerable. He was admitted to the Sorbonne in 1843, although the examiner for his entrance chemistry examination labeled him mediocre. It was in his last year, while he was working on his doctoral dissertation, that serendipity gave Pasteur its first gift. It happened in this manner.

It had been known for a few years that tartaric acid existed in two forms, although their atomic constitution was identical. One form was able to rotate the plane of polarized light to the right, whereas the other type was totally unable to do the same. This distinction of course mystified chemists; they could not understand why these two forms of tartaric acid, absolutely identical in number and character of atoms, reacted so differently to polarized light.

Pasteur, on a hunch, decided to examine the crystals of the tartaric acid that had no power to change the direction of polarized light. This was the serendipitous gift—but it was his perceptive mind that noticed that this form of dried tartaric acid comprised two different sorts of crystals. The differences were slight, but to his sharp eyes quite distinct. With a small tweezers he collected each form in separate tubes of pure water. When he placed the first vial before the source of polarized light, the light was rotated to the right. The tube of water containing the second variety of crystals turned the light to the left.

He thus had made two major discoveries. First, he had isolated a previously unknown tartaric acid, one that turned polarized light to the left. Second, and more important, he had determined why one of the two tartaric acids was unable to rotate polarized light at all: it was composed of crystals that turned polarized light in opposite directions and therefore neutralized each other.

This tremendously significant finding, described by a twenty-five-year-old chemist in a doctoral dissertation,[4] raised Pasteur to instant recognition and fame. His discovery essentially gave birth to the science of stereochemistry. Immediately after the discovery, he was appointed to the professorship of chemistry at Dijon. When he was appointed professor at Strasbourg in 1849, he married the woman who remained with him for the rest of his long life.

It was not until 1857 that Pasteur left the world of lifeless chemical substances and their reactions to enter the invisible but living world of minuscule plants and even tinier animals—Leeuwenhoek's world. Two aspects of this exotic microscopic world simultaneously absorbed his attention.

The first was the bitterly debated but still obscure matter of spontaneous generation. The concept of living things arising from inanimate substances appeared so ridiculous to Leeuwenhoek that in 1702 he wrote in one of his letters to the Royal Society, "Seeing these wondrous dispensations of Nature whereby these 'little animals' are created so that they may live and continue their kind, our thoughts must be abashed and we ask ourselves, can there even now be people who still hang on to the ancient belief that living creatures are generated out of corruption?"

Despite this early-eighteenth-century assertion that spontaneous generation should be a dead issue, it continued to flare for well over a century after Leeuwenhoek's death. Not even the distinguished studies of Lazzaro Spallanzani in 1765 or those of Theodor Schwann in 1839—demonstrating that the growth of living organisms, ordinarily easily occurring in meat broth, would not take place if the broth mixture was boiled and then sealed against the entrance of air—were effective in stilling the claims of some investigators. They continued to insist that putrefaction always was due to organisms arising de novo from decaying dead animal or plant tissues.

It is very doubtful that Pasteur had ever heard of Leeuwenhoek, much less read his 1702 article in the *Transactions of the Royal Society*. But he had known of Schwann's 1839 experiment. (Characteristically, Pasteur failed to refer in any of his articles to Schwann's earlier work, but in a private letter he did acknowledge the pioneering, indeed crucial, findings of Schwann.) He also was aware of the objections of those who criticized the experiments of both Spallanzani and Schwann. They insisted that these two men, by sealing their broth mixtures *after* boiling them, had prevented the ingress of air. It was their belief that there was some gaseous but nonliving element in the excluded air that was necessary for the emergence of living organisms from nonliving elements.

Pasteur therefore drew out the open tops of glass tubes containing meat broth and narrowed them to a small diameter. The narrowed tube tips were directed downward so that the openings, while permitting the entrance of air, barred the ingress of heavy particles that might be suspended in the air.

Such broth mixtures were boiled to kill any microorganisms and then incubated. They uniformly failed to show putrefaction or growth of any kind.

Pasteur's simple experiment should have destroyed the concept that living matter sprang from nonliving materials. But the concept of spontaneous generation persisted in the minds of a few investigators until the clear-cut, definitive studies of the bacterial nature of air particles by the English physicist John Tyndall in 1876–1877.

Pasteur was still engrossed in his studies relative to spontaneous generation when he was importuned by French beer makers and vintners to determine what was ailing their processes—a serious matter indeed in a country so devoted to both beverages. It was during these studies that Pasteur found that the fermentation process on which the production of both beer and wine depended was brought about by various yeasts. Again, Theodor Schwann several decades earlier had demonstrated the existence of living and reproducing yeasts and was fairly certain that they were responsible for the production of alcohol from barley. A full half-century before Schwann's discovery, old Leeuwenhoek had described yeasts and the globules they produced.

Pasteur did more than discover the significance of certain yeasts in the fermentation of beers and wines, however. He found and demonstrated methods of preventing the deposit and growth of the stray airborne yeasts that had so seriously injured the beer and wine industries. From his studies arose the idea of gently heating fluids to destroy possible contaminating yeasts and bacteria, a process today called pasteurization and universally used for the preservation of various food products.

Having saved the beverage industries of France, Pasteur hoped that he could return to his laboratory and resume his studies of chemicals and their reactions with one another. But that was not to be. He was prevailed on by one of his former teachers to investigate a malady that was decimating the silkworms responsible for one of the chief rural industries of France. Perhaps he would have escaped being pressed to enter a field of study that was entirely foreign to him if he had not been insisting since 1863 that all putrefying processes were caused by microorganisms, and that it was putrefaction, pure and simple, that was destroying the small silkworms.

During the five years he devoted to an investigation of the sickness killing the silkworms, he never was able to identify the germ that he was certain was responsible. He *was* able to devise methods of quickly detecting the illness in the silkworms, and by meticulous isolation and hygienic methods prevent the spread of the disease and ultimately eliminate the epidemic.

As the savior of the beer, wine, and silk industries, Pasteur by 1870 was the most revered scientist in France, perhaps in the world. Exactly what occupied him after he had saved the silkworm industry in 1870 is not quite clear. There is no question, however, that his interest shifted from chemistry to Leeuwenhoek's little animals.

Although Pasteur was not a physician, he managed to visit the morgues of hospitals, taking particular interest in women who had just died of childbirth or puerperal fever. He certainly knew of the studies of Ignaz Semmelweis and Oliver Wendell Holmes, who had cleverly demonstrated that this fever was contagious. Unlike the two physicians, Pasteur obtained samples of the blood of the uterus and its exudates from the corpses of Parisian mothers who had just died of puerperal fever. When he microscopically examined the various samples and took cultures, he always found one of Leeuwenhoek's little animals, a microorganism that appeared to be composed of a series of tiny beads (which now are designated streptococci).

Pasteur never published a single word describing these findings, and they would not be known to us except that he lost his temper one evening in March 1879, while listening to an obstetrician give a lecture on puerperal fever at the Paris Academy of Medicine. When the speaker sneeringly dismissed the idea that a microbe caused the disease, Pasteur interrupted and yelled, "The cause of this disease is doctors who carry a germ from a sick patient to a healthy one." The speaker retorted that such a microbe would never be found. Pasteur bounded from his seat and went to a blackboard, saying as he did so, "I shall show you the microbe." And he drew a small chain of beadlike structures on the blackboard. The incident was never published, but how proud Leeuwenhoek would have been at hearing of it!

In 1878 Pasteur turned his attention to the organisms causing chicken cholera, and serendipity again bestowed a precious gift. Uniformly, when he injected chickens with a culture of the cholera germs, the animals died within twenty-four hours. But one day he injected two chickens with a culture that was not fresh, but was several weeks old. The two chickens promptly became sick but recovered; Pasteur instructed his assistant to put them back with the healthy chickens.

The entire laboratory staff at that time was excited about an upcoming vacation. When the holiday ended, they resumed injecting chickens with the usual fresh cultures of cholera. Along with all the other chickens, the two that earlier had survived being injected with the aged culture received an inoculation of the deadly fresh culture. All the chickens died the next day—except the two that had previously survived. Unlike the lifeless corpses of their fellow chickens, they were lively and well.

When Pasteur saw the two gamboling about and briskly pecking at their food, his mind was ready to take advantage of this second great favor that serendipity had bestowed on him. Indeed, his mind was overwhelmed by these two chickens, whose survival had opened the path that would ultimately lead to the saving of millions of unborn children and adults. He was dazzled because he instantly recognized that he had made the greatest discovery of his life. Furthermore, Pasteur at first fantasized that the injection of an *aged or weakened* culture of cholera germs would not only protect an animal from a later infection of cholera, it also would offer protection from all other diseases.

After a few months of fevered, overenthusiastic, but consistently disappointing study of other diseases, the reality manifested itself: injection of an animal with an old culture of cholera germs afforded future protection to this animal against cholera, and only cholera. Pasteur, confronted with this specific limitation of his discovery, quickly recognized that just because injection of weakened cholera germs offered no protection against other diseases, the injection of weakened germs of other diseases would not necessarily be worthless in protecting against the diseases that these germs caused. It was this insight that gave birth to bacterial vaccination.

Pasteur at this critical juncture had almost certainly read of Koch's brilliant discovery two years earlier that the anthrax bacillus caused anthrax. So Pasteur knew two facts: first, that anthrax was caused by a germ, and second, that at least as far as cholera was concerned, a chicken injected with an attenuated culture of cholera germs protected that chicken forever against an attack of cholera. Might not, he reasoned, the same protection against *anthrax* be afforded an animal who had been inoculated with an age-weakened culture of anthrax bacilli?

His hunch proved to be correct. He found after many trial-and-error studies that if cultures of anthrax bacilli were carefully attenuated by aging, they *generally* could protect an animal against a second injection of a lethal culture of anthrax bacilli. Prolonged, meticulous study was needed to find a foolproof method of developing attenuated cultures of anthrax bacilli that were too weak to kill or seriously weaken recipients on injection, but powerful enough to provide immunity to a later injection of lethal anthrax bacilli.

The precautions required patience and time—and Pasteur was not a patient man. Although he found that usually he could afford protection against lethal injections of anthrax bacilli, such was not invariably the case. Occasionally the inoculation of a supposedly attenuated culture led to the death of the injected animal.

Despite these admittedly infrequent "misfires," Pasteur prematurely revealed in late 1880 that he had found a vaccine that could protect sheep and cattle from anthrax. Challenged in the spring of 1881 by a committee to provide a public demonstration of the efficacy of his anthrax vaccine, Pasteur immediately accepted. The event was to take place at Poilly-le-Fort on May 31–June 2. Just how concerned Pasteur was with meeting this challenge will never be known, but we believe it likely that he was very much involved in the technical preparations.

On May 5, 1881, Pasteur and his assistants inoculated twenty-four of forty-eight sheep, three of six cows, and one of two goats with cultures of attenuated anthrax bacilli. These same animals were reinjected on May 17. Then on May 31 all the preinjected as well as the uninjected animals were inoculated with a lethal culture of anthrax bacilli. The crucial demonstration was held on June 2, at which time distinguished physicians, members of the press, and scores of other interested spectators assembled to observe the results of the deadly injections given on May 31.

On June 1 Pasteur received a message stating that some of the vaccinated sheep given the deadly culture the day before already were becoming ill. Tense and emotionally overwhelmed, Pasteur turned on Pierre Roux, his loyal colleague, and in violent, bitter language accused him of performing the preliminary vaccinations in a sloppy, careless way. "I will not go tomorrow to be humiliated because of your mistakes in vaccinating the sheep. You have made this horrible mistake, now you go by yourself tomorrow to face the jeering crowd," Pasteur is said to have screamed at him in an uncontrollable frenzy. Fortunately his wife was present and managed to calm him down somewhat. But it was not until late in the evening of the same day, when a telegram arrived announcing that all the vaccinated sheep were doing well, that Pasteur decided to take the train to Pouilly-le-Fort.

When Pasteur and Roux arrived, they knew from the cheers of the crowd that greeted them that their experiment was successful. At the demonstration field they found twenty-two of the sheep that had not received the vaccine lying dead on the ground; the two remaining control sheep were dying. The twenty-four vaccine-protected sheep appeared totally normal as they grazed unconcernedly. The cow and the goat that had not received the vaccine lay dying or dead on the field; but the cows and goat that had received the vaccine were completely well.

It was a magnificent triumph for Pasteur. He became again a national hero, and an international one besides. Within days he was besieged by thousands of sheep and cattle growers for his magical anthrax vaccine, and hundreds of vials of the vaccine were sent from his laboratory. Pasteur and his assistants were overwhelmed by this international deluge. Pasteur had not perfected a system of preparing the vaccine that ensured its nontoxicity as well as its potential to provide immunity to the animals injected with it. Soon, many instances occurred in which the vaccine injection killed the sheep and cows, or in other instances failed to provide protection against the later onset of anthrax.

Because of the frequent mishaps, Robert Koch, smarting because Pasteur had never referred to his own seminal anthrax studies, began publicly to criticize both the cholera and the anthrax studies of Pasteur. Stung by these criticisms, coming as they did just a few months after his successful anthrax vaccine demonstration at Pouilly-le-Fort, Pasteur violently attacked Koch at the Fourth International Congress of Hygiene and Demography, held in Switzerland in 1882.

After Pasteur had finished his polemic, the chairman of the congress invited Koch to respond. In his most insulting manner, Koch replied that he had come to the congress to learn something new about the attenuation of bacteria, but he had learned nothing. He refused to respond to Pasteur's remarks because he did not believe that the convention was the correct place for such a debate—and also because he did not speak French well and Pasteur did not speak German at all. He promised that he would respond in the proper medical journals to Pasteur's criticisms and point to errors in Pasteur's studies (which he proceeded to do in more than one journal). Pasteur responded scathingly that Koch would have learned many new facts at the congress if he had understood the French language.

Koch in the ensuing publications pointed out that the administration of Pasteur's anthrax vaccine often killed the animals it was supposed to protect, and that the inoculations too often failed to prevent the onset of anthrax, particularly in sheep. Aware of these dangerous inconsistencies, Koch had examined some of Pasteur's vials of supposedly pure culture of attenuated anthrax bacilli. He found that often the cultures were contaminated with bacteria other than anthrax, and frequently the anthrax bacilli were insufficiently attenuated and lethal. These findings of course pointed to the shoddiness and haste with which the vaccines were prepared.

The published statement that created a permanent hostility between these two giants was in one of Koch's papers criticizing Pasteur's methods and his means of announcing and demonstrating his anthrax vaccine. The last sentence read, "Such goings-on are perhaps suitable for the advertising of a business house, but science should reject them vigorously." As we shall see, however, Koch proceeded in the same fashion in 1890 with the introduction of his tuberculin.

Despite Koch's biting criticisms, Pasteur was able to repeat his Pouilly-le-Fort demonstrations of the efficacy of his anthrax vaccine in 1882 in Germany itself. Given this triumph, his earlier achievements in founding the science of stereochemistry, and his salvation of the wine, beer, and silk-producing industries of France, Pasteur, now sixty years old and partially crippled by an earlier stroke that had weakened his left leg, could have rested on his laurels and done what modern investigators do when they reach that age—become an administrator.

Instead, he began in 1882 to study the vicious and always fatal disease, rabies. It is believed that he chose to investigate this disease because he was never able to forget an early childhood experience of seeing heated, flesh-burning irons applied to the bite wounds of a child attacked by a mad dog. Whatever his motive for taking up this malady, it presented a terrible danger to him and his assistants. Their experimental animals were rabid dogs, and initially the only way of studying the disease was to house a normal dog with a rabid dog so that the sick animal could transmit rabies to the normal dog by biting it repeatedly.

Pasteur guessed that he was studying a disease caused by some minute germ, even though he had found no such entity despite repeated microscopic attempts. Even with a microscope equipped with the newly invented Abbe condenser and an oil immersion lens, this infectious agent (which we now know is a virus) was not then and is not now detectable.

Observing a delay between the time a human or an animal was bitten and the onset of symptoms of rabies, and noting that these symptoms arose chiefly from a disturbed brain and spinal cord, Pasteur cleverly concluded that the infectious agent must travel via the peripheral nerves to concentrate eventually in the brain and spinal cord. This assumption would later prove to be of tremendous importance.

Pasteur and his assistants had been working for several years on this wretched disease when serendipity again intervened. Its gift this time was a dog. Although it became rabid after being bitten by another dog with rabies, this dog did what no other rabid dog had ever done: it recovered completely. Furthermore, when injected with fresh brain tissue from a rabid dog, which Pasteur previously had found invariably led to rabies, the dog remained totally free of the disorder.

This marvelous chance occurrence was not lost on Pasteur. He began to inject spinal-cord tissue obtained from rabbits who had been infected with rabies. Except that he first gave spinal-cord extracts attenuated by letting them age for a number of days before they were injected. His scheme worked! He inoculated dogs each day with spinal-cord extracts (obtained from rabid rabbits), beginning with an extract that had been dried and set aside for fourteen days and then injecting on each succeeding day an extract set aside one day less. After many trials he found that by the fourteenth day the dogs could receive fresh cord extract—which if given initially would invariably have sickened them with rabies—and fail completely to show symptoms of the disease.

Unlike his hurried, impatient production of anthrax vaccine, Pasteur proceeded cautiously in these experiments. By 1885, three years after beginning his work on rabies, he was reasonably sure that his system of injecting, over a period of several weeks, increasingly less attenuated rabies-infected spinal-cord extracts would provide complete protection against rabies.

Then, one day in 1885, a distraught French mother brought her son to Pasteur, begging him to save the boy. Two days earlier he had been bitten severely fourteen times on his arms, legs, and thighs by a rabid dog. Pasteur was not a doctor; nor was he sure that the prophylactic treatment that had given immunity to his injected dogs would do the same for nine-year-old Joe Meister. He sent the boy to two physician friends who were aware of his laboratory studies. When these doctors saw the festering bite wounds, both of them urged Pasteur to administer his therapy to the child. Pasteur agreed to give the boy daily injections for thirteen days of cord extract of continually increasing lethality. This regimen required great courage on Pasteur's part, knowing as he did that the extract given on the thirteenth day would inevitably have been lethal if given on the first day. But the child was saved, and news of this great victory spread instantaneously throughout the civilized world. (When the Pasteur Institute was founded, Joe Meister became its custodian for the remainder of his long life.)

A few weeks later, nineteen Russian peasants who had been bitten two weeks earlier by a rabid wolf came to Pasteur for his therapy. He injected each of them twice a day for seven days. All Paris was alerted to this dramatic fight against death from rabies. When sixteen of the peasants were saved, the Russian Czar was so appreciative that he sent Pasteur the diamond cross of Sainte Anne, together with 100,000 francs to be used for construction of a Pasteur Institute.

Within several years, extracts were prepared by laboratories in various countries. Deaths due to rabies almost disappeared. Although initially in 1885 Koch had sneered at this method of prevention, within a year he too began to employ Pasteur's method of preparing the extracts.

This awesome medical feat was Pasteur's last. In 1892, for his seventieth birthday, he was honored with a special medal before an extremely distinguished audience. Limping badly, he was escorted by the president of the French Republic. He was too weak to give his own speech, and it was given by his son. He died in 1895 holding a crucifix in one hand and his wife's hand in the other.

Not many contemporary high school graduates would recognize by name the majority of scientists described in this book. But every single one would recognize and identify Pasteur as probably the greatest of all scientists. Very, very few of these youngsters would know of his founding of stereochemistry, or of his discovery of anthrax vaccine — but all would recognize the process bearing his name, pasteurization. And perhaps a goodly fraction would recognize him as the developer of the antirabies vaccine.

Without question, Louis Pasteur was France's most distinguished scientist. Frightfully egotistical, reluctant to give credit to his predecessors or his contemporaries, sometimes a bit dishonest, an unabashed showman, and (paradoxically) a bitter foe of physicians — still, it is not likely that France will ever again nurture a scientist of such unparalleled elegance.

Of course, old Leeuwenhoek would have admired and sometimes been irritated by Pasteur's pioneering but theatrically presented findings. He would also have been hurt and angered by Pasteur's complete omission of Leeuwenhoek's own seminal discoveries, as well as those of virtually all other investigators who had preceded him. Nonetheless, this 1673 observer of the heretofore invisible little animals would have been overwhelmingly impressed, if more than two hundred years later, he had found himself in an amphitheater at Breslau, surrounded by some of Germany's most distinguished professors, watching and listening to a short, thirty-three-year-old, darkly bearded, round-faced country physician from an obscure Prussian village. This man was demonstrating for the first time in the history of medicine that one of Leeuwenhoek's little animals, the anthrax bacillus, was the cause of a disease that attacked not only animals but humans too.

No, not even Pasteur was the first to demonstrate that one of the little animals could cause human disease. The obscure, unprepossessing general practitioner — Robert Koch — had spent three years employing only a microscope and a few hand-fashioned tools, had worked in a curtained-off space in his consultation room with only his medically untrained wife as an assistant, had isolated the anthrax germ from sick animals, had cultured it, and had observed it change into what he called spores, which were capable of surviving indefinitely under the most unfavorable circumstances. Finally, he had injected cultures of this same bacillus into guinea pigs and other animals, including sheep and cows, and observed that when they promptly died, their bodies were riddled with this terrifying new enemy of both man and animal.

The famous German professors Ferdinand Kohn and Julius Cohnheim, who were in this hastily called ad hoc assembly in Breslau to observe for three successive days the demonstrations of this nonacademic country doctor, were totally awestruck at what was being revealed. So impressed were the two academicians that they determined that the unknown doctor had to be rescued from medical obscurity in Wollstein. But first they must publish the astounding discovery that a tiny bacterium could cause a human disease. Six months after the June demonstration at Breslau, Kohn published Koch's anthrax studies in the journal he himself edited.[5] Kohn and Cohnheim worked until 1880 to get Koch appointed to the Imperial Health Institute in Berlin. There for the first time he was given a decent laboratory and two skilled assistants and was totally freed from general medical practice. He did not even have teaching duties.

Koch continued his research activities at Wollstein during the four-year interval that elapsed between his first anthrax discovery and his move to Berlin. It is difficult to determine whether he consciously was aware during this period that he was preparing himself almost exclusively (discovering and fashioning new techniques and instruments) to make the greatest bacteriological discovery that the world would ever know. What is known with certainty is that during these four pre-Berlin years, he worked with the optical experts Ernst Abbe and Carl Zeiss and probably was the first scientist to equip his own microscope with their light condenser and their oil immersion lens. It was the fitting of his microscope with these two optical inventions that allowed him to visualize bacteria that previously were incapable of being seen because of their small size. Also, sharper and more exact morphological details of Leeuwenhoek's little animals could now be observed. Koch also took advantage of new aniline dyes of various sorts. Some bacteria could be stained by one dye but not by others, and Koch used this property to differentiate species of bacteria.

One day Koch happened to notice a cut potato that had been exposed to the air for several days. What he saw intrigued him: there were raised spots of different colors on the surface of the potato. When Koch excitedly examined these spots, he observed that each was composed of microorganisms. Moreover, the microorganisms of a given spot were all identical, but were different from those of another spot of a different color. To an ordinary person this serendipitous observation would be at best mildly interesting. To Koch, desperately seeking a way of obtaining pure cultures of different species of bacteria, it led to an immediate recognition. If instead of dipping a drop containing various bacteria into a *liquid* culture medium (which at the time was the uniform way of culturing bacteria), he were to gently smear the same tiny drop across a *solid* culture medium, the various species of bacteria in the drop might form separate colonies on the surface of the solid medium and thus isolate themselves from the other bacteria in the drop.

It did not take Koch long to find that the addition of gelatin to the usual broth employed to grow bacteria resulted in a solid broth medium. When he lightly brushed the surface of a solid broth plate with a tiny loop that had been immersed into a broth containing various species of bacteria, the next day—after the solid broth had been placed in an incubator—he found discrete but often colored spots dotting the surface of the plate. He observed that each bacterium of any given spot or color growing on the surface of the gelatin-broth plate was exactly the same as the remaining bacteria of this same colony, but possibly different from other colonies on the plate. Koch must have felt gloriously enriched, because by this relatively simple maneuver he would be capable of isolating and growing a pure culture of any bacterium he wished—a feat no one else had ever accomplished. The importance of this feat to his later studies in Berlin will shortly become evident.

Koch had only been at the Imperial Health Institute in Berlin for thirteen months before he began in absolute secrecy what was to be his outstanding medical contribution: discovery of the bacterium that caused tuberculosis. Why did Koch in August 1881 tell no one that he was trying to find the germ that caused tuberculosis? Perhaps the main reason was that only five years had passed since his article on anthrax had demonstrated unequivocally that a bacterium was the cause of a disease that attacked human beings as well as animals. Prior to his anthrax work, almost no one believed that any of Leeuwenhoek's little animals could cause human disease, particularly tuberculosis. Even after the anthrax discovery, medical luminaries such as Rudolph Virchow and Theodore Billroth still denied the possibility that living microscopic animals were responsible for any disease. Indeed Virchow, when told by the young Koch that adaptation of the oil immersion lens to a microscope permitted the visualization of bacteria heretofore invisible, replied that anything not seen by his present microscope was not worth seeing.

Further, Koch himself was not at all sure that tuberculosis was caused by a bacterium. Even if one were responsible, would it be too small to see? Would he be able to stain it?

Then too, would he be able to grow such a bacterium in pure culture so that he could inject it into animals to demonstrate that his bacterium produced the same disease as the one in nature? No one knew better than Koch that it was his injection of the anthrax bacillus into animals, and its reproduction of anthrax in those animals that convinced most of the scientific world in 1876 that he had made an outstanding medical discovery.

Faced with these potentially insuperable difficulties, Koch had only an essentially intuitive belief that if a bacterium caused anthrax, he would find a different bacterium that caused tuberculosis.

Finally, he kept his work secret even from the other members of the Imperial Health Institute because if he were to identify and demonstrate a bacterium that caused tuberculosis, he wanted Robert Koch and no one else to get the glory. He was as intent on becoming famous as was Pasteur and even before commencing his tuberculosis studies, Koch planned to surpass Pasteur in terms of worldwide fame. Then too, since the Franco-Prussian War the fiery, flamboyant Pasteur had made no secret of how much he detested Prussians; Koch, a prototypical Prussian, had little or no tolerance for a peasant Frenchman, which is what Pasteur really was.

In a method similar to that of his earlier anthrax studies, Koch began to search for the suspected tuberculosis bacterium in tubercular tissue of human subjects overtaken by the disease. The tubercle, the characteristic pathologic lesion present in the lungs of consumptive patients, was the tissue he subjected to the various new aniline dyes. He then searched for a specific bacterium with a microscope that was five times more powerful than even the best of Leeuwenhoek's hundreds of instruments.

Koch took only a month or less to find that by staining a section of a tubercle with methylene blue dye, he could detect in all tubercles a tiny, rod-shaped bacillus, much smaller than the anthrax bacillus. He called it the tubercle bacillus. If his microscope had not been equipped with its oil immersion lens and condenser, he never would have found the bacillus.

Koch realized that detection of the tubercle bacillus in the tubercles of diseased patients was only the first step in his search for the cause of this dreadful disease. He properly reasoned that perhaps the germ he saw was a secondary parasite growing in tissue previously damaged by some other agent. Obviously, he must isolate and grow the bacillus in pure culture and then see if injecting it into animals would produce tuberculosis.

As he had learned to do when working with anthrax, he rubbed bits of diseased tissue over the surface of solidified agar, hoping that in the next day or so discrete colonies of the bacillus would develop. No such luck! What did these wretched bacilli require to grow? Koch must have pondered that question dozens of times as he failed repeatedly to obtain a pure culture. Then, with incomparable vividness of imagination, he decided to offer the recalcitrant bacteria a medium that might feel more like a human or animal body. He added blood serum to his agar and lightly smeared infected tissue over this serum-rich agar surface.

Once again there were no bacterial colonies to be seen in twenty-four, forty-eight, or even seventy-two hours of incubation of the media. Since all previous bacteria had grown profusely in twenty-four hours, Koch might well have thrown away the serum-agar plates. But Koch did no such thing. He remembered that tuberculosis, unlike other human diseases, rarely proved fatal in weeks or even in months. So why should not the suspected bacillus grow slowly? Koch asked himself. He continued to incubate his cultures for weeks, peering daily along the surface of his serum-agar plates.

At the end of several weeks, his patience was rewarded by the appearance of tiny grayish-white colonies. He quickly scooped up a bit of one of these colonies with his platinum loop, smeared the contents on a glass slide, stained it, then examined it with the oil immersion objective of his microscope. To his intense satisfaction, he observed millions of tubercle bacilli—and only tubercle bacilli. He had succeeded in obtaining for the first time a pure culture of just one species of bacteria.

Having obtained this pure culture, Koch took the next critical step: he injected healthy animals with pure cultures of his suspected tubercle bacillus. Invariably such animals sickened after a week or so, and when sacrificed always exhibited bodies decimated by typical tuberculosis lesions. When Koch took tiny bits of the lesions from these animals, stained them, and examined them with his microscope, he observed that they swarmed with myriad tiny, thin rods—exactly the same as the rod-shaped microbes he consistently detected in human tubercular tissues.

"Now I can truly call this microbe the tubercle bacillus, because I see it and only it in all human tubercles. I have grown it in pure culture, I have inoculated animals with pure cultures of it, and these animals always became tuberculous. Finally, I find the same bacillus in their diseased tissues," glowed Koch, who by nature was not an emotional man.

When Koch inoculated his animals with a pure culture of a bacterium originally obtained from human tuberculous tissue, and those animals sickened and died of tuberculosis, he knew his discovery was one of the most magnificent ever made in medicine. He also knew that even though he had just passed his thirty-eighth birthday, he would become one of the most famous medical scientists in the world when he announced this monumental scientific revelation. But first, he cautioned himself, he must announce this discovery, made after less than seven months.

Koch revealed his discovery on March 24, 1882, at a meeting of the Berlin Physiology Society. The small meeting room was packed with Berlin's most celebrated physicians, because rumors had circulated for several weeks that Koch was going to announce a major discovery. At the end of his detailed account of the steps he had taken to prove that what he called the tubercle bacillus was the cause of human tuberculosis, every physician in the room was stunned. Their amazement stemmed in part from the innovative procedures—the use of aniline dyes, the addition of potassium salt to the dyes, the employment of solidified culture media, the methods for obtaining pure cultures, and the patience in finally getting the tubercle bacillus to grow in the test tube—that Koch had had the brilliance to invent. But the physicians were more than amazed, they were awed by the emotionally and intellectually unexpected revelation that would forever change their concept of what caused so many human diseases. Indeed, this evening meeting had witnessed the birth of bacteriology. Paul Ehrlich, who later would discover a cure for syphilis, was at the meeting. Remembering it years later, he exclaimed, "That evening has remained my greatest experience in science."

The discovery was published less than three weeks after Koch's talk.[6] As he had anticipated, his announcement catapulted him to a fame as great or even greater than that of his French rival, Pasteur. Instantly world renowned, Koch was besieged by bright young scientists eager to learn his techniques so that they might identify the germs causing other diseases. It was not too long before Koch's followers isolated the tetanus and the diphtheria bacilli, and developed antitoxins that would protect against the ravages of these two diseases.

The years after the 1882 discovery were exciting, satisfying ones for Robert Koch insofar as his scientific career was concerned. However, his relationship with Emmy, his wife, became intolerable to both of them. We probably shall never learn what embittered these two persons, both of them still relatively young. Most likely he neglected her, so fascinated and engrossed had he become with his researches. Then too, it can be disastrously unsettling to a scientist who has won the admiration and respect of all the civilized world to return nightly to be treated as an ordinary husband who is expected to perform his usual chores about the house. It probably was difficult also for a proud German wife of fifteen years to adulate continuously, without a hint of criticism, a husband who was far from ideal. Most scientists are not receptive to domestic criticism, and Koch certainly was far from tolerant or easygoing in his home environment.

In any event, when their only child, a daughter, married in 1888 and left their home, Koch and Emmy no longer lived together. Was he upset or relieved by the separation? We suspect, in view of what later took place, that he was relieved. Ever since Emmy had presented him with the microscope on his twenty-eighth birthday, he had found science to be an alluring mistress who had given him first the ineffable joy of discovering some of the secrets of nature, and then the even more enticing gift of lasting fame. So he worked harder and longer in his laboratory, and made additional minor discoveries until 1890. Then Koch stumbled, and he stumbled badly.

The disaster began at the Tenth International Medical Congress, a prestigious assembly hosted by Germany. For the general sessions, Berlin offered its largest auditorium, which seated eight thousand persons. It was before this huge audience of the world's preeminent scientists that Koch would duplicate what he had scathingly accused Pasteur of doing: killing instead of protecting thousands of animals with a hastily produced vaccine. But at this 1890 meeting, what Koch was to say would lead to the premature deaths of hundreds of human beings.

Even before he made his self-damning and dishonest speech, he was aware that the German government craved that he announce something to dazzle this assembly of renowned scientists in the same way as his announcement of the bacterial cause of tuberculosis had stunned the world eight years earlier. Here was an audience to whom to proclaim that he, an official of the German imperial government, had discovered a probable cure for tuberculosis. After all, this imperial government had already informed him that in the very next year it would build a new institute that would bear his name and be devoted solely to the study of infectious diseases. What if he very cautiously hinted obliquely that he had found "substances" that did seem to be *hopeful* in combating tuberculosis in a few of his guinea pigs. The young Koch, the meticulous Koch, the completely truthful Koch, would never have finished a talk to the Tenth International Medical Congress with this essentially false sentence: "In spite of past failures, I continued the quest and I ultimately found substances that halted the growth of tubercle bacilli not only in the test tube but also in animal bodies."

Even as he made this statement, he knew that his data were far too incomplete to warrant it. So in his very next sentence he said, "My only reason for departing from my usual custom, by reporting investigations that are not yet complete, is to provide incentive for additional attempts in this area." It was a generous sacrifice of his former integrity, ostensibly to stimulate others to find a cure for this disease. In actuality, this second sentence was no more honest than the first, because scientists in reality seek only one prize: priority of discovery. Rarely are they noble enough to bend their efforts to inspire other scientists to enjoy the intense excitement stemming from being first. And although Koch possessed some incomparable traits as a scientist, nobility was not one of them.

The first sentence quoted above was transmogrified within days by the newspapers of the entire world into a declaration that a cure for tuberculosis had been announced by the renowned German scientist Robert Koch. Again, as Pasteur had been besieged a few years previously by thousands of sheep and cow growers intent on obtaining his anthrax vaccine, so Koch in turn was overwhelmed by tubercular patients and their physicians to obtain what he called tuberculin—the protein he had extracted from the tubercle bacillus. Within a few months hundreds of thousands of consumptive patients were given Koch's tuberculin in the hope that it would halt the progress of their disease. Because tuberculosis often does disappear as a progressive disease, when this happened in persons who had been given Koch's tuberculin, the subsidence of the acute symptoms was attributed to tuberculin.

Controlled experiments carried out in various laboratories, however, failed to confirm the therapeutic efficacy of Koch's wonder drug. Further, it soon became apparent that injections of tuberculin worsened the course of tubercular infection in hundreds of patients. In a ghastly echo of Pasteur's wild haste to distribute his anthrax vaccine, Koch repeated the same mistake, thereby killing hundreds of tubercular patients. Nor did it help that he engaged in an acrimonious public confrontation with a former student, Adolph von Behring, who wished to patent his own supposed cure for tuberculosis.

The German government went through with its construction of the Koch Institute for Infectious Diseases, despite the waning prestige of its still-eminent scientist. It was in 1893, while sitting for his portrait to be installed in the Koch Institute that Koch, with nothing else to do, happened to notice a small portrait of a very beautiful, very young woman. Koch could not take his eyes from this beguiling face. Emmy, separated from him, had never been beautiful and now in her late forties she no longer attracted Koch. He must encounter this new lovely person, three decades younger than his own fifty years! Perhaps his fame would dazzle her sufficiently that she could forget the vast difference in their ages. He determined to make an all-out effort to pursue and conquer her.

The artist painting his portrait told him her name, Hedwig Freiburg, and that she was a part-time art student, a bit player in the theater, and unmarried. Koch's pursuit of her was hectic, ardent, and quickly successful. They were married in the same year, 1893, a few months after his divorce from Emmy.

Most medical historians have been inclined to assume that the social ostracism that followed Koch's marriage to the twenty-one-year-old Hedwig caused him great discomfort and sorrow. However, we do not believe that Koch, having found "a thing of beauty," missed one whit the repetitious routine of sitting at formal dinners next to the often-frumpy wives of the academicians and bureaucrats who made up his social world.

If Berlin society as he experienced it bored him, his research still fascinated him. And his lifelong, wistful desire to visit strange and exotic countries took on an irresistible attraction after his new marriage. Thus, from 1893 until his death in 1910, Koch journeyed almost continuously to different parts of Africa and India, seeking out possible means of eradicating sleeping sickness, cholera, malaria, and intractable infections that killed cattle and sheep. He was almost always accompanied in these travels by his young wife. In the last several years of his life, he journeyed to the United States and Japan—not to study some mysterious disease, but to bask in the acclaim and adulation he expected these two great nations to shower upon him. He was not disappointed.

Still, his pride received a bitter blow when the first Nobel Prize in Medicine was awarded in 1901 to his former student and later his bitter enemy, Adolph von Behring. His own pioneering achievements in bacteriology, though, were too magnificent to be ignored because of his tragic error in falsely announcing the curative power of tuberculin. In 1905, Robert Koch too received the Nobel Prize.

Koch began to experience symptoms of coronary heart disease and suffered a myocardial infarction in 1910. Hoping to recover from this attack, he went to Baden-Baden with his wife. But he died shortly after his arrival.

Other than Hedwig, only ten persons attended his burial; and there were eleven wreaths. Pursuant to his wishes, no priest officiated at the ceremony. Georg Gaffky, an investigator of some stature, was the only scientist attending the funeral. He spoke for several minutes and a dirge followed. The entire ceremony was over in six minutes.

Robert Koch was not a noble person, not a particularly pleasant man. The absence of these two qualities partially explains why this true father of bacteriology has failed to become a distinguished hero of medicine. No great cinema or stage play will ever illustrate his life; brilliant as were his achievements in the laboratory, Koch was essentially a dull man. But the dull man was obsessed with one goal: to find which of Leeuwenhoek's little animals caused which diseases. In discovering the little animals that caused anthrax, and the little animals that caused tuberculosis and cholera, Koch founded the science of bacteriology. He is the scientist Leeuwenhoek would have admired most. Of one thing we are certain: we shall forever be indebted to the general practitioner of Wollstein, as we shall be to the haberdasher of Delft and to the eccentric Frenchman.

4

Edward Jenner and Vaccination

Even the most casual students of English literature are aware of Lady Mary Wortley Montagu's association, both pleasant and later viciously unpleasant, with Alexander Pope. Probably they are also aware of her surpassing beauty. But very few of these students are aware of the circumstances that led to her striking the first blow against smallpox, a blow that made it possible for Edward Jenner, long after she died, to discover the means that has wiped this disease from our planet. Before we examine Lady Mary's actions and why she took them, let us first describe smallpox itself.

Smallpox was a ghastly illness. An apparently normal person would suddenly become desperately sick, develop a high fever, headache, backache, vomiting, and delirium. On the third or fourth day red spots would appear on the skin, changing in a few days to blisters that filled with pus.

Most of these terrible lesions occurred on the face (even the eyes), but also on the forearms, hands, legs, and feet. If the patient survived, scabs would form and fall off over the next few weeks, leaving pitted scars that would remain indefinitely.

Smallpox epidemics killed 20 to 40 percent of the people who developed the disease, and those who lived were dreadfully disfigured or even blinded. During the seventeenth and eighteenth centuries, one-third of the entire population of London bore the horrible scars of smallpox, and two-thirds of blind people had lost their sight because of smallpox.

In 1980, though, this scourge disappeared forever. The number of people infected with smallpox gradually declined over a period of two centuries, after Edward Jenner introduced vaccination, one of the ten supreme discoveries of Western medicine.[1]

Physicians had long looked for cures. Healers in ancient China and India observed that one attack of smallpox conferred "lifelong" immunity. (We now know that in some cases immunity lasts many years, but it is not necessarily lifelong.) They conceived the idea that causing a mild attack of smallpox might prevent a full-fledged attack later on. So they ground to a fine dust a smallpox scab taken from a survivor, then using a silver tube blew this dust into one of the nostrils. If the subject was a man, the dust was blown into the left nostril; if a woman, into the right nostril. The person then would usually but not always develop a mild case of smallpox, even if the dust was as much as six months old. Upon observing these preventive measures, an English trader, Joseph Lister, wrote to a Fellow of the Royal Society, exhorting him to implement the technique in England; but the Fellow was unimpressed.[2]

In the meantime, the Arabs had developed a different method. They made small cuts in a healthy person's arm and rubbed into the incision material obtained from a smallpox blister. A famous Turkish physician living in Constantinople, Dr. Emmanuel Timoni, was so taken with this method that he wrote a book in English describing it in detail. He tried unsuccessfully to distribute it in England in 1715, but the book made no impact on British physicians. This Turkish physician, Dr. Timoni, will reappear shortly in our account. For now, let us return to Lady Montagu and her role in eliminating smallpox.

Lady Mary Wortley Montagu, until 1717 at least, was triply blessed.

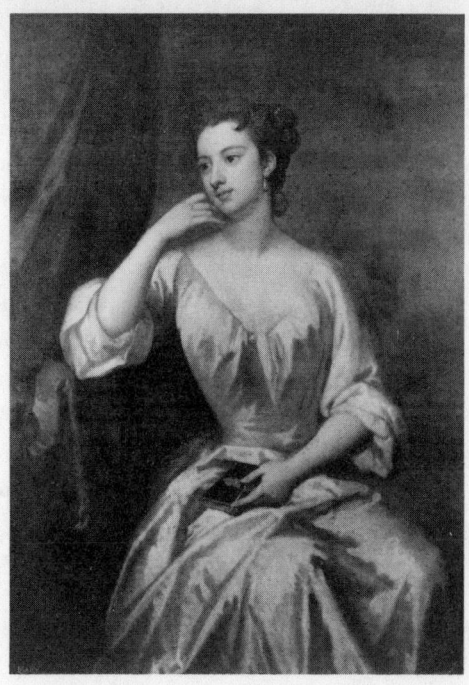

FIGURE 5. Lady Mary Wortley Montagu, as painted
by England's distinguished artist Sir Godfrey Kneller.

She was of the noblest blood, her father being the Duke of Kings-
ton. She was so beautiful that England's most celebrated painter of the
time, Sir Godfrey Kneller (who had painted fourteen sovereigns, including
Charles II, Louis XIV, and Peter the Great), eagerly sought to paint her
and succeeded in capturing her beauty on canvas (see Fig. 5). Alexander
Pope, on first seeing it, was so impressed that he wrote a poem whose first
few lines declare:

> That happy air of majesty and
>   truth,
> The equal lustre of the
>   heavenly mind,
> Where every grace with every
> Virtue's joined.

Nobly born, lovely of face, Lady Montagu's third blessing was brilliance of mind. All three were hers until 1717, when she contracted smallpox while living in Constantinople with her husband, who served as England's ambassador to Turkey. Although she survived the smallpox, her face was disfigured with many ugly, ineradicable scars that no cosmetic could completely hide. She who had delighted in looking into mirrors now shunned them.

In this same year, 1717, she gave birth to a daughter. Her English physician, a Dr. Maitland, fortunately for unborn generations of mankind, called in Dr. Timoni to assist him in the delivery. Timoni, immediately noticing that Lady Montagu's face was badly scarred, persuaded her to allow him to immunize her first child, a son. Lady Montagu agreed, and when both Maitland and the Montagus returned to England, Maitland immunized the young daughter he and Timoni had delivered.

The Latin for smallpox is *variola*, so the new procedure became known as variolation. Lady Montagu wished to publicize it, so she invited three members of the Royal College of Physicians of London to visit her daughter after her inoculation at the hands of Dr. Maitland. These members, in turn, insisted that Sir Hans Sloan, the president of the college, support variolation. He agreed to do so, albeit very reluctantly. Lady Montagu, who had a nose for public relations, also invited newspaper reporters to the first variolation in England, which received widespread publicity.

Although the approval of the Royal College of Physicians and the dramatic newspaper stories might persuade the public to accept variolation, Lady Montagu knew that a further step would be required: she had to convince royalty of the need to variolate their own children. Accordingly, she approached Princess Caroline of Wales with the suggestion that she variolate her two daughters. The princess responded that she needed further evidence that the procedure was safe, so Dr. Maitland did what was common practice in those days; he experimented on six prisoners, who were subsequently released, and a young orphan. The seven successful outcomes satisfied the princess that the procedure was safe and could be used on her own children.

By 1735, some 850 people in Britain had undergone variolation. The numbers remained small because some surgeons had introduced a preparatory period, for which there was absolutely no rationale. For six weeks prior to variolation, they bled their patients, placed them on a low-calorie diet, and purged them vigorously. Not surprisingly, by the end of this six-week regimen all the patients were thin and weak. It would be thirty years before surgeons would finally abandon this barbaric ritual. In the meantime, the members of the Royal College unanimously decided to lend their strongest support to the new technique of variolation.[3]

Its results were not as uniformly positive as the early reports indicated. Modern estimates suggest that about 12 percent of those treated died, an extraordinarily high figure that would be totally unacceptable today. Compared to the alternative, however—a mortality of 20 to 40 percent during a severe epidemic—variolation was the lesser of two evils. Since its success was only relative, variolation never became popular in the American colonies and in fact was outlawed by several states.

Clearly, a safer way of preventing smallpox was urgently needed. The person destined to develop that method, Edward Jenner, was born in Berkeley, Gloucestershire, near Bristol, on May 17, 1749. His father, Stephen, had become a clergyman in the Church of England. He married Sarah Head, daughter of the Reverend Henry Head, Vicar of Berkeley, and became Vicar of Berkeley himself after Head died.[4]

Stephen and Sarah had nine children, two of whom died; Edward, the eighth child, became an orphan at the age of five years. His mother died at age forty-six, following the birth of her ninth child, and his father died two months later, at the age of fifty-two.

Because his two eldest brothers, Stephen and Henry, were studying at Oxford, his three sisters, Mary, Sarah, and Ann, looked after the young orphan. But it was with Stephen, who also became a clergyman and who guided him throughout his youth, that the young orphan bonded and for whom he had a deep and grateful affection. Edward loved music and became quite an accomplished violinist and flutist. One of his neighbors, an older boy, Thomas Beddoes, later would play a notable role in the history of vaccination.

When Edward reached the age of eight years, his brothers and sisters decided to send him to a free boarding school. An event occurred there that was to leave an indelible impression on the young Jenner: a terrible smallpox epidemic. All schoolchildren who had not yet undergone variolation were required to do so, including Edward. In this strange environment, the young orphan found himself subjected to the useless and potentially dangerous preparatory ritual of bleeding, fasting, and purging. Six weeks later, extremely weak, emaciated, frightened, and miserable, he was inoculated, then confined with other children who had contracted smallpox, most of them desperately ill.

This frightful experience had serious psychological consequences for Edward, among them severe anxiety, insomnia, and auditory hallucinations. Realizing that he was in trouble, his older brothers and sisters decided to send him to a very small private school, where he was able to make a number of lasting friendships. His closest friend, Caleb Parry, later participated in some of Jenner's developed medical interests.[5] But the curriculum (Greek, Latin, and religion) did not suit Edward's temperament or innate abilities. He was a poor student of Greek and Latin and became bored and disinterested. Fortunately, he developed two outside interests, raising doormice and collecting fossils.

Stephen and Henry had hoped that Edward would follow in their footsteps to Oxford, but the entry requirements were strict: an excellent background in Greek, Latin, and religion. Someone (probably Stephen) had sufficient sensitivity and insight to realize that Edward's interest lay in biological phenomena and suggested that a career in medicine might be more suitable for him.

Edward could not qualify for the best medical schools of the time, either—Oxford or the Scottish medical schools. Although changes were beginning to occur in the British medical system, the division between physicians and surgeons still existed. Surgeons, who were much less educated, acquired their medical knowledge through apprenticeship rather than academic work at one of the universities. The College of Physicians was a Royal College, the College of Surgeons was not. Physicians were addressed as "Dr.," surgeons as "Mr."

Although undistinguished, Edward's academic achievements qualified him for training as a lowly surgeon. English children of all classes in the eighteenth century often assumed adult responsibilities at a much younger age than now. Surgeons, for example, hired remarkably young apprentices. Jenner was scarcely thirteen when he was apprenticed to a country surgeon, John Ludlow, with whom he trained for six years. While working for Ludlow, he enjoyed listening to the anecdotes country folk told their surgeon. One tale he heard in 1768, toward the end of his training, was that milkmaids who caught cowpox on their hands never caught smallpox later. Cowpox was a harmless disease of the udders and teats, only affecting cows in Britain and Western Europe. Hearing these stories first gave Jenner the idea that deliberately giving people cowpox might prevent them from catching smallpox later.[6]

Before Jenner could investigate his idea further, he moved to London, where he enrolled as a student at Saint George's Hospital. At the time, the hospital was neither well known nor respected, but its chief of surgery, John Hunter, would soon build a reputation as the most outstanding surgeon in England. Hunter had decided to rent rooms in his house to his students, and Jenner was his first boarder.

Jenner became the closest friend Hunter ever had, yet their personalities were completely different. Hunter was an exaggeratedly rough Scotsman, impatient, impolite, arrogant, domineering, and overcritical. Jenner, the younger man, was kind, caring, considerate, polite, and scrupulously honest. Hunter found Jenner's calm manner soothing, while Jenner frequently referred to Hunter as "that dear man." Realizing that anyone who criticized or disagreed with Hunter could raise his ire, Jenner went out of his way to protect him, aware that Hunter had begun to suffer from what was then a mysterious and eventually fatal disease, angina pectoris.

No other British medical school could have provided the unique education Jenner received during his two years at Saint George's. He gained considerable experience in the latest surgical techniques; more important, he learned from Hunter not to speculate, but to prove or disprove a hypothesis by performing a well-conceived experiment. This concept is taken for granted today, but in the eighteenth century it was still a relatively novel idea. Also, a new science known as physiology had appeared on the horizon. Although Hunter had always considered anatomy important, he had begun to realize that physiology was its equal.

Over time Hunter had acquired a collection of some thirteen thousand anatomical, pathological, and biological specimens (which later became the foundation of the Hunterian Museum). Because of Jenner's knowledge of this collection and his expertise in classifying specimens, Hunter recommended him to Captain James Cook when Cook returned to England aboard the *Endeavour* in 1771. Jenner was to classify the thousands of plants Cook's chief botanist, Sir Joseph Banks, had brought back. Jenner did such an outstanding job that Banks invited him to accompany Cook on his second voyage around the world, but Jenner declined. Even Hunter could not persuade him to go. After two years in London, Jenner longed for the peace and quiet of the English countryside. He had never had any real family life, and he desperately wanted to return to Berkeley and be near his eldest brother, Stephen, of whom he was so fond.

Long before his stay in London, indeed ever since his medical apprenticeship, it had been cowpox, always cowpox, and how it probably conferred immunity against smallpox, that had been on Jenner's mind. He discussed his thinking with Hunter many times, sketching for him the typical cowpox lesions involving the hands. Hunter was so impressed that he always mentioned the association between cowpox and immunity to smallpox in his lectures to students. One of them told a visiting physician, Joseph Adams, about this theory. Adams, in turn, pointed out the possible association in his famous book, *Observations on Morbid Poisons Chronic and Acute*.[7]

Soon after Edward Jenner went back to Berkeley, because he had gained quite a reputation in London he began receiving very attractive job offers to return to that city. Hunter begged him to come back and become his research assistant, an offer he apparently felt Edward could not refuse. The University of Erhalenken, hoping to attract him there, wished to confer an honorary doctorate on him. Another group promised an enormous salary if he would join a surgical practice in India. All these offers Jenner politely but firmly declined; his roots were in Berkeley, and he refused to be uprooted.

Wealth in Berkeley was measured in land, and the wealthy automatically became the local gentry. By these standards Jenner, who had by this time inherited a large amount of land and property, was a country gentleman. His avocations—music, writing, viewing great works of art, ornithology, and chemistry—were as important to him as his vocation. Local people frequently referred to him as "the adventurer." Everyone enjoyed his company because he was fun loving, talented at playing the violin and flute, charming, imaginative, and curious. Friendships were extremely important to him and he remained in constant contact with school friends.

Skilled in the social graces and busily engaged in a country medical practice, Edward Jenner continued to remain in close communication with his London mentor, John Hunter. It was probably at Hunter's suggestion that Jenner began his studies of the cuckoo in the 1780s.

Long before Jenner began to investigate this strange bird, it was known that the cuckoo never built a nest of its own, never hatched its own eggs, and never fed the newly hatched cuckoos. Why this fantastic bird deposited its eggs for hatching in the nests of common hedge-sparrows was unknown. Even more mysterious was the fact that within twenty-four hours of the nestlings' emergence from their shells, all the eggs or nestlings of the host hedge-sparrow that had been in the nest were ejected. Jenner resolved to find the explanation of these almost eerie phenomena.

Studying the migration cycle of the cuckoo, he discovered that, unlike other birds visiting England, the cuckoo did not appear there until after mid-April and did not produce its eggs until after mid-May. The eggs required at least two weeks of incubation before the nestlings emerged. Then the nestlings remained in the nest for two to three weeks before attempting to fly and search for their own food. Jenner discovered that by July first all cuckoos had migrated from England. Cuckoo offspring were deserted before they had learned to fly and forage for themselves.

Jenner was satisfied that he had solved the mystery of why the cuckoo left the incubation of her eggs and the nourishment of her offspring to the hedge-sparrow. Unlike the cuckoo, which arrived in England too late in the spring and departed too early in the summer, the hedge-sparrow would remain in England to perform her instinctual duties. Exactly how nature encouraged the female cuckoo to choose the hedge-sparrow as a substitute, Jenner did not try to explain. He did discover, by patient, continuous observation of many hedge-sparrow nests containing a cuckoo egg or nestling, exactly how the host's own eggs and nestlings disappeared from her nest less than a day after the cuckoo egg had hatched.

To his great surprise, Jenner noted that within an hour of the cuckoo's hatching, and despite its weakness and total blindness, it began to search the nest for other nestlings or eggs. Jenner was even more astounded when he observed that the cuckoo nestling was employing the tips of its wings as a searching tool. If another nestling or still unhatched egg was detected by the roving, searching wing tip, the cuckoo nestling would slowly approach the detected egg or nestling, then scoop underneath it. Having secured the prey in a peculiar depression in its back, the young cuckoo would lift it to the top of the nest, then with a convulsive, jerking movement eject the egg or nestling. Several times Jenner, having observed this macabre expulsion, would replace the nestling in its nest. But the searching wing tip would detect the returned nestling and eject it once more.

Jenner happened to come upon a nest in which two cuckoo nestlings had just been hatched. We will let Jenner's own words describe what happened:

> In just a few hours after their hatching, a contest began between the cuckoos for the possession of the nest, which continued undetermined till the next afternoon, when one of them turned out the other. . . . The contest was very remarkable. The combatants alternately appeared to have the advantage, as each carried the other several times nearly to the top of the nest, and then sunk [sic] down again, oppressed by the weight of its burden, till at last after various efforts, the strongest prevailed and was afterwards brought up by the hedge-sparrow.

After having observed these oddities, Jenner examined the backs of cuckoo nestlings to discover the nature of the depression there that allowed the nestling to securely carry and finally eject from the nest an egg or nestling. Again, we employ his words for this description:

> The singularity of its shape is well adapted to its purpose; for, different from other nestlings, its back from the scapula downwards is very broad, with considerable depression in the middle. This depression seems formed by nature for the design of giving a more secure lodgement to the egg of the hedge-sparrow or its young one, when the young cuckoo is employed in removing either of them from the nest. When it's about twelve days old, the cavity is quite filled up and then the back assumes the shape of nestling birds in general.

Knowing that John Hunter was interested in stomach hair balls of various animals, Jenner also examined the stomachs of quite a number of cuckoo nestlings and was happy to discover some hair balls there. He dispatched them to Hunter, who was positively delighted to add them to his rather grisly collection. In fact, Hunter was so pleased with Jenner's cuckoo researches and the resulting hair balls for his precious (to him) museum collection that he had Jenner describe all his cuckoo findings in a letter to him. He had this letter published in the *Philosophical Transactions of the Royal Society* in 1788.[8] The paper created a sensation and was responsible for Jenner's subsequent admission into the Royal Society.

Jenner did not spend all his time carrying on a countryside medical practice and observing cuckoos. He found time to play both the violin and the flute, as well as compose ballads and songs. When he learned that 18 million African blacks had been transported to the Western Hemisphere by 1772, he was so shocked by the size and inhumanity of the slave trade that he wrote the music and lyrics for an antislavery song:

> If, when me nothing had to eat,
> For stealing bit of bread,
> Black man you so severely beat,
> And whip till almost dead;
> What Punishment's to Massa due?
> From Guilt can he be Free?
> Who, when he bought poor Negro, knew
> That white man steal a me.

In addition to these avocational activities (assuming that the practice of medicine was his vocation), when Jenner heard that two French brothers had flown a passenger-carrying balloon filled with hydrogen, he forthwith himself constructed a large balloon of silk, filled with hydrogen. Although never a passenger on a flying balloon, this country doctor was the first person in the British Isles to produce a passenger-carrying flying balloon. Each stage of the process was equally enjoyable to him: building the balloon, manufacturing the hydrogen to inflate it, doing the scientific experimentation, and savoring the successful outcome. (Soon afterward, passenger-carrying balloons became popular in the United States, where Benjamin Franklin was one of the first Americans to fly in one.)

An eligible gentleman of Jenner's stature naturally attracted the attention of many young women, but despite his social charm and grace, he found it difficult to establish a meaningful relationship. Hunter knew that Jenner did carry on a love affair with a young woman, an affair that ended after about ten years. Jenner never told anyone who the woman was, and her identity remains a mystery to this day. After the romance fell apart, he was extremely depressed. His preoccupation with ballooning lifted his spirits, as did his involvement with another woman, Catherine Kingscote, who lived in a village of the same name established by her family. In order to impress Catherine, and no doubt her influential family, the flight of Jenner's second balloon began in Kingscote. It must have been successful, because on March 6, 1788, Edward married Catherine in the Kingscote parish church. He was thirty-eight, she twenty-seven. Edward, who had courted Catherine for several years, had anticipated the nuptials and bought a cottage in Berkeley.[9]

No two people could have been more different; it was a case of opposites attract. She was an introvert, had few friends, and disliked social gatherings and parties. She had only three interests: Edward, religion, and (after they were born) her children. Nevertheless, she was a good woman who tried to cater to all Jenner's needs, even reluctantly giving large parties when he asked her to do so. Perhaps most important, she left him free to pursue both his vocational and avocational activities.

All the while, Jenner never lost his interest in a baffling disorder first described by William Heberden in 1772. He called the illness angina pectoris. Heberden described the symptoms of the disorder and recognized that eventually it was lethal; but he had no idea of what went wrong in the chest to produce the characteristic pain felt by patients. Nor did Jenner or Hunter immediately determine the cause when Hunter, with Jenner looking on, performed an autopsy in 1772 on one of Heberden's patients who had died suddenly while experiencing the disorder. Jenner recalled that although Hunter looked at the heart of Heberden's patient during the autopsy, he did not examine the coronary arteries.

Some time after 1783 and before 1793, Jenner himself was performing an autopsy on a patient who had died while having an attack of angina pectoris. Jenner, describing the autopsy in a letter to his good friend Caleb Parry, wrote:[10]

After having examined the more important parts of the heart, without finding anything by means of which I could account either for his sudden death or the symptoms preceding it, I was making a transverse section of the heart pretty near its base, when my knife struck against something so hard and gritty, as to notch it. I well remember looking up to the ceiling, which was old and crumbling, conceiving that some plaster had fallen down. But on further scrutiny the real cause appeared: the coronaries were becoming bony canals.

This finding of calcification of the coronary arteries first made Jenner suspect that it was obstructive disease of those arteries that was responsible for angina pectoris, and for the sudden death that so often occurred in the course of the disorder. His suspicion became a certainty after further autopsies of patients dying of angina pectoris revealed that such patients invariably possessed one or more severely obstructed coronary arteries.

Jenner at the time of this discovery knew that his mentor and dear friend, John Hunter, was suffering from angina pectoris. He did not want Hunter to know that the cause of his angina was the ominous obstruction of one or more of his coronary arteries. Therefore he decided not to publish this tremendously significant discovery. Never before in the history of medicine had an important discovery been withheld because of the friendship of one man for another, and the desire to avoid inducing sadness in the friend.

While Jenner did not inform Hunter of his coronary findings, he did tell the physicians treating Hunter of his observations, but they made light of them. After Hunter died in 1793, however, one of his physicians examined the coronary arteries at autopsy and reported to Jenner that he had been correct: Hunter's coronary arteries were severely obstructed.

Intrigued and involved as he had become in such disparate subjects as the behavior of the cuckoo nestling and the cause of angina pectoris, Jenner still remained intrigued by the possible relationship of cowpox to horsepox and human smallpox. At a medical meeting he met a Mr. Frewster and learned that Frewster had in 1765 presented to the London Medical Society a paper on cowpox and its ability to prevent smallpox. (The paper was never published.) Frewster's account of a possible relationship between the two diseases fascinated Jenner. As a result, he and Frewster so dominated the medical society's meetings with discussions of the various poxes that members of the society threatened to expel Jenner if he persisted. They insisted that the topic could have no medical relevance.

Today we know that smallpox, cowpox, swinepox, horsepox, and a large number of other animal poxes are caused by orthopox viruses and that all

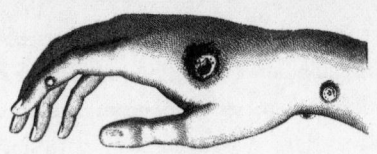

FIGURE 6. This drawing, which shows
the pustules on the hand and wrist of
a milkmaid suffering from a cowpox
infection, appeared in Edward Jenner's
1798 book describing the protective power
of cowpox vaccination against smallpox
infection.

such diseases can infect humans (see Fig. 6). An infection with one member of the disease group immunizes a person against infection with all the other members. This last fact Jenner did not know, but when a historic event occurred in December 1789, Jenner immediately recognized its transcendent importance.

A nurse who had looked after Edward Jr. subsequently developed swinepox. Two other women also had been in contact with the infected nurse. On December 17, Jenner took samples from the nurse's swinepox lesions and inoculated all three people (his son as well as the two women who had been exposed) with this material. On the ninth day after inoculation, all three became ill and developed a few raised red lesions where Jenner had made the incisions on their arms.

A few weeks later, he variolated all three with smallpox; none developed symptoms or a rash. Although Jenner did not realize it, this was a truly memorable occasion. He had taken material from a person with swinepox, had inserted it into three healthy people, and in this way had protected them against smallpox.

On July 18, 1790, a Dr. Hicks informed the Gloucestershire Medical Society that there had been an outbreak of swinepox in that community. Jenner discussed his experiment with Hicks, and at the September meeting of the society they jointly read a detailed paper on Jenner's experiments on his son and the two women who had been exposed to swinepox. This historic paper produced little reaction from the audience because no one present recognized its true significance. Jenner himself remained cautious and variolated his son with smallpox again in December 1790. Edward Jr. later had a typical smallpox reaction, albeit a mild one. We now know that swinepox confers only temporary immunity against smallpox. Still uncertain, Jenner variolated Edward Jr. a third time with smallpox in December 1791. That time there was no reaction whatsoever. Predictably, smallpox had protected against smallpox for a longer period of time than swinepox had.

For the next several years, Jenner apparently experimented no further on the poxes. He contracted typhoid fever in 1795 and during his slow convalescence resided at Cheltenham, a famous spa. As he relaxed there—possibly while bathing in the spa, although we shall never know for certain—he devised a brilliant experiment, essentially similar to the one he had already conducted on Edward Jr. and the two women. His new research plan was simple enough. He would inoculate a normal person who had never had smallpox, with cowpox. After that person had recovered, he would variolate the subject with smallpox; if the smallpox variolation did not take, it would mean that cowpox had conferred immunity against smallpox.[11]

Jenner could not keep a secret, so he surely must have discussed his proposed experiment with many people. In the meantime, more clinical examples of cowpox protecting against smallpox were surfacing, adding to his confidence that the experiment would succeed. Since cowpox had a tendency to disappear after a few years and then suddenly reappear, Jenner realized his scheme would work continuously on a large scale only if he transmitted cowpox from human to human. He would have to choose his experimental subject carefully, so that the subject's family would not initiate a public outcry if anything went awry. He selected an eight-year-old boy, James Phipps, whose father, a homeless laborer, worked for the Jenners. Sarah Nelmes, the daughter of a prosperous farmer, served as the donor; a thorn scratch on her hand had become infected when she milked a cow called Blossom that had cowpox.[12] Jenner had no qualms about the experiment. After all, human cowpox was a mild disease from which no one had ever died.

The eventful day finally dawned: May 14, 1796. Jenner made two incisions, each one-half inch long, on James's left arm. After dipping the point of his lancet in the fluid obtained from Sarah's cowpox lesions, he inserted it into the two incisions. Eight days later, pustules similar to those seen after cowpox appeared. For the next two days, James had a slight fever. On the ensuing July 1 Jenner variolated James, which should have given him an attack of smallpox. But as Jenner had predicted, James did not develop the slightest sign of the disease. For the first time in history, Jenner had unequivocally demonstrated that giving a normal, healthy person cowpox — a very mild disease in humans — protected that person against smallpox, and that human-to-human transmission of cowpox could easily be accomplished.

At last a safe method existed for eradicating smallpox from the face of the earth, although it would take two centuries to achieve that goal. Clever as Jenner's experiment was, its validity rested on the fact that smallpox did not appear after James had been variolated. We wonder what Lady Montagu's reaction would have been to Jenner's discovery that cowpox vaccination provided protection against smallpox. We believe she would have been very proud of the fact that she had introduced variolation in England, because Jenner's discovery was in large part due to the fact that cowpox vaccination prevented variolation from producing its usual smallpox!

Exciting and provocative as the case appeared to be, Jenner knew that he had to consolidate his apparent victory against this killer of many millions. He had foresightedly obtained fluid from the innocent pustule that James had developed following his inoculation with cowpox. Jenner inoculated a second group of patients with drops of James's fluid; when these patients developed cowpox pustules, he withdrew fluid from them to inoculate another group of patients, and inoculated subsequent groups by the same means. In this way he was able to inoculate eight children, aged eleven months to seven years. Two of the seven were later variolated, with negative results. One additional child was not inoculated with cowpox but was variolated instead. That child did react, indicating that the material used for all four variolations was potent. Seven of the eight young people who were inoculated with cowpox reacted to the inoculation; all seven were children of laborers or workhouse inmates.

Jenner had such faith in the cowpox inoculations that one of the eight children was his own son, Robert. Ironically, Robert's inoculation was the only one of the eight that did not take. Shortly after inoculation, a smallpox epidemic broke out, so Jenner did what any father would do under the circumstances — he variolated his own son.

Jenner spent July and August feverishly preparing a paper for publication. Traveling to London, he submitted his paper to Sir Joseph Banks, president of the Royal Society, for publication in *Philosophical Transactions.* Jenner had every confidence that it would be published. Sir Joseph had the very highest regard for Jenner's abilities, and it was he for whom Jenner had catalogued thousands of plants collected on Captain Cook's trip. It also was Sir Joseph for whom Jenner had done a meticulous experiment proving that manure was a better plant fertilizer than human blood. But it was Sir Joseph who decided unilaterally to reject Jenner's paper, even though two manuscript reviewers had strongly recommended publication. He said that Jenner needed more cases, and that he ought not to risk his reputation by presenting a learned body with something so much at variance with established knowledge.

Jenner realized that to prove his point convincingly he needed to repeat his experiment on at least a few more subjects. But as luck would have it, cowpox disappeared for the next two years. Jenner did not just sit and wait, however. He prepared multiple copies of a new paper, which he distributed to his five most trusted friends, asking them to advise him of any necessary modifications. This de facto editorial committee met on March 1, 1797, and offered its suggestions, one of which apparently was that Jenner should publish his valuable material privately. Later that year he visited London again and made arrangements to do just that.

After Jenner had succeeded in accumulating a few more cases, he returned to London. There he worked frantically to revise his original manuscript.[13] Dedicating this seventy-five-page book to his lifelong friend Caleb Parry, Jenner himself paid for the printing. When it appeared in 1798, its cost was only a shilling; today a copy would fetch $25,000. (And it *should* cost that much, not just because it has become a relatively rare book, but also because it gave birth to the only method medicine has yet devised to *prevent* the onset of an infectious disease—whether the disease is rabies, bubonic plague, or poliomyelitis. Perhaps also AIDS?)

The thrust of the message carried by Jenner's small book was that cowpox could protect persons against smallpox. Unlike variolation, vaccination with cowpox was safe. No one died from and no one was wretchedly scarred by cowpox. Also, occasionally the smallpox induced by variolation was contagious, whereas cowpox appearing in the human after inoculation with cowpox fluid induced in the human a mild disorder that was never contagious.

Far in advance of his time, Jenner further suggested in his book that cowpox diseases were caused by a "virus"—obviously not a virus in the modern sense, but some kind of infectious principle. He adapted a word that had been used in English since about 1590 to mean a poison.

Jenner in his book described exactly how he performed the cowpox inoculation. His technique was so effective that it remained the standard for the next two hundred years. He also pointed out that he had based his paper partly on clinical experience, partly on research, partly on a hypothesis. Finally, he promised to continue his research, because he believed it would benefit humanity. Nowhere in his book did the name of Lady Mary Wortley Montagu appear.

With the success of his book, Jenner now had the opportunity to make himself instantly wealthy and famous. Henry Cline, his friend and chief of surgery at Saint Thomas Hospital who had begun giving cowpox inoculations, offered him 10,000 pounds a year to relocate his practice to London. Jenner declined. Commenting in a letter to a friend that he had enough money, he vowed that at no point would he attempt to enrich himself through his discoveries.

Jenner soon realized that pure cowpox vaccine was not easy to obtain, preserve, or transmit. Although the relationship between bacteria and infection had not yet been discovered, he warned of the dangers of using putrefied material, and eventually discovered that it was best to remove fluid from a human cowpox lesion between the fifth and the eighth days. If it was removed earlier, it was ineffective; but if later, it could cause what we now call a secondary bacterial infection.

Within a short time Jenner published two more pamphlets,[14] one of them again dedicated to Caleb Parry. Translations of his various writings soon appeared in Europe. In 1800 Jane Austen wrote that she had attended a dinner party at which her host and hostess read Jenner's pamphlet on cowpox. It was not only the medical profession that had become interested in Jenner's work! It should come as no surprise, therefore, that by 1800 even the King of England had heard of Jenner's work. On March 7, 1800, the Earl of Berkeley presented Jenner to the king, who granted him permission to dedicate the forthcoming second edition of *An Inquiry into the Cause and Effects of Variolae Vaccinae* "To the King."

An etymological advance occurred in 1803, when the word *vaccination*, derived from the Latin word *vaccinia*, meaning cowpox, replaced the clumsy descriptive phrase *cowpox inoculation*. Richard Dunning, a surgeon in Plymouth, England, who had performed a large number of vaccinations, coined the term.

Soon after the publication of Jenner's original book, physicians and surgeons began vaccinating people, initially in London and Gloucestershire, but almost immediately also in the rest of the British Empire, Europe, the United States, and eventually the world. In July 1800 Daniel Waterhouse, aged five, son of Dr. Benjamin Waterhouse, professor of the theory and practice of physics at Harvard University, was the first U.S. citizen to be vaccinated. Dr. Waterhouse became an ardent advocate of vaccination and successfully urged President Thomas Jefferson to support it. Within a few years several thousand people had been vaccinated in London alone. Henry Cline got the ball rolling. Two other physicians George Pearson and William Woodville, however, did not make Jenner's life easy.

Pearson surveyed a large number of physicians and surgeons familiar with Jenner's *Inquiry*, publishing the results of his survey as "An Inquiry Concerning the History of Cowpox Principally with the View to Supersede or Extinguish the Smallpox" in November 1798. All the responses strongly favored vaccination, and Pearson gratefully acknowledged the contribution Jenner had made to its discovery.[15]

Pearson then did something that required Jenner's immediate attention: he founded the Institute for the Inoculation of the Vaccine-Pock. The first Jenner heard of the matter was when Pearson sent him an invitation to attend the inauguration and to become an ordinary member of the institute. Jenner was shocked. Clearly, Pearson was attempting to take credit from him. Jenner refused to join or attend the inauguration unless he was put in charge of the institute. When Pearson did not agree to this demand, Jenner lobbied a large number of influential people, who boycotted the institute. All this political activity took a great deal of time away from Jenner's research, writing, and family.

Woodville, a physician in a smallpox hospital, in May 1799 wrote a pamphlet called "Report on a Series of Inoculations for Variolae Vacciniae with Remarks and Observations on this Disease, Considered as a Substitute for Smallpox." This report, based on Woodville's extensive experience, confirmed Jenner's work. But immediately after publication, a number of patients he had vaccinated developed rashes all over their bodies. Pearson then had a similar experience with his own patients at the same hospital. Woodville subsequently published a pamphlet called "Observations on the Cowpox," which attacked Jenner's assertion that vaccination causes a rash limited to the vaccination site. Pearson published a similar article in the *Physical and Medical Journal* in 1800.

Jenner, upset by these damaging reports, insisted that what had happened was that the cowpox vaccine had become contaminated with smallpox vaccine. He even sent Woodville samples of pure cowpox vaccine to prove his point. Neither conceded that the other was right; throughout this scientific disagreement, Jenner exhibited his too-pronounced characteristic, stubbornness. His unwillingness to compromise in the slightest degree unnecessarily lengthened the debate and increased its intensity.

A Dr. Benjamin Moseley was another thorn in Jenner's side. He wrote a treatise in 1799 referring to vaccination as "cowmania." He mocked Jenner's work, calling cowpox *lues bovita*, or cow's syphilis. Developing the analogy further, Moseley suggested that, like syphilis, cowpox might eventually affect the brain.[16]

A report by William Rowley, M.D., claimed that one child had developed an ox-faced deformity a year after vaccination and that a girl had developed mange (a skin disease seen in hairy and woolly animals) following her vaccination. Drawings of the two children appeared in the article, suggesting that the cowpox vaccination would inflict animal diseases on humans, or turn them into animals. As late as 1808, Richard Reese, M.D., published his *Practical Dictionary of Domestic Medicine*, in which he attacked vaccination and listed the names of numerous physicians who disapproved of it as well.

Naturally Jenner had his supporters too. One of the staunchest was John Ring, a surgeon at Saint Thomas Hospital. Ring placed a full-page advertisement in favor of vaccination, signed by many of the leading physicians and surgeons in London, in the *Morning Herald* of July 19, 1800, and published numerous articles disputing the claims of those who opposed vaccination.

The general public gradually became aware of all the adverse opinions about vaccination. Jenner's premonition of a fame pierced with the arrows of malignancy was coming true. Somehow or other, in the midst of the hostile criticism, Jenner managed to remain calm and confident. There were small cracks in his armor, however; he occasionally remarked that he showed his friends everything but his back.

Jenner also recognized that for the remainder of his career he would be unable to devote sufficient time to his wife and children, and the realization worried him. Orphaned at the age of five, he knew only too well what the lack of family life could mean to young children. His private practice had begun to suffer from his long absences in London and the time he spent on research, writing, and politics. After a few years he actually bought a house in London because he found himself spending several months a year there.

By this time Jenner was generating very little income from his practice. The situation became genuinely serious: he was more than 12,000 pounds in debt, a huge sum in those days. He realized full well that he had erred in telling Cline that he did not need money. He decided to establish his own private practice in London. Unfortunately for him, most potential patients realized that vaccination was a simple procedure that their own surgeon or physician could easily perform, so he failed to build a practice.

He and his supporters hit on the idea of submitting a petition to the British Parliament, asking its members to grant a reward to compensate him for the expenses incurred while working on vaccination. They tried mightily to secure the success of the petition, while he returned to Berkeley to await the outcome. There he found his wife in a very poor state. Suffering from tuberculosis, she had become depressed and had turned to religion for help, so much so that a friend warned Jenner that both his sons might become clergymen. Nor was this a time of marital harmony; Catherine disapproved strongly of his petition to Parliament. She argued that he should keep to his original plan of living off his own income, which was sufficient for their needs—so she thought.

The House accepted the petition, the king approved it in principle, and a Committee of the House examined witnesses for about a month. After subjecting Jenner to intense interrogation, they called numerous witnesses both for and against vaccination. Interestingly, one of Jenner's strongest supporters was Thomas Beddoes from the Pneumatic Institute in Bristol. He had become convinced of the efficacy of vaccination after its results had so impressed the medical community in Bristol that they considered presenting an award to Jenner.

As one would expect, the strongest opposition came from Birch, Moseley, and Pearson. Pearson insisted that he and Woodville had vaccinated many more people than Jenner had and that they, therefore, deserved priority. Pearson knowingly lied: he told the committee that it was he and Woodville, not Jenner, who had discovered that it was safe to vaccinate infants.

In the end, the House agreed to grant Jenner money; the only point of contention was how much. Various members proposed 20,000 pounds, 15,000 pounds (either of which would have solved Jenner's financial problems), or 10,000 pounds. After much debate they unanimously voted, on June 2, 1802, to grant him a reward of 10,000 pounds.

Jenner's colleagues and friends recognized his achievements by honoring him in other ways. In 1802 Guy's Hospital Physical Society named him an honorary member. The Naval Medical Officers gave him an award for saving so many lives during the Napoleonic War, and the Royal Jennerian Society was formed. As the title would indicate, the king and queen were his patrons and their children vice patrons, with over fifty of the most influential people in Britain at the helm. They published scientific reports and provided free vaccinations for the poor. At its first scientific meeting in 1803, the Royal Jennerian Society officially approved the term *vaccination*. And on August 11, 1803, the City of London granted Jenner freedom of the city, presenting him with a gold box worth 105 pounds that contained the certificate. A month later the Royal Humane Society made him an honorary member.

Now an "old" man of fifty-four years, nationally and internationally famous for his work, admired for his political and social skills and status, but still as poor as a churchmouse (he owed more than 2,000 pounds even after the parliamentary award), Jenner sold his house in London in August 1803 and returned to Cheltenham and Berkeley. There he reestablished his practice and there he remained for the next two years.

Both Jenner and his wife were very sympathetic to the poor. At the time, the gentry, a very small percentage of the population, owned all the property in England and had the vote all to themselves. Even though the Jenners were in debt, his deeply religious wife spent much time with the local poor. Jenner himself built a clinic adjacent to his cottage, which he called the Temple of Vaccinia, at which he gave free vaccinations.

There can be no doubt that without Jenner's continued personal effort and his political skill during the ensuing years, vaccination would not have become firmly established in medical practice. While in Cheltenham, he continued his vigilance in this respect, noting with sadness that those physicians, surgeons, and apothecaries who opposed vaccination were gaining ground. Fewer people were vaccinated and more were variolated. As a result, more than eight thousand people died of smallpox in London in 1805. Much of Jenner's time was devoted to letter writing in defense of the cause of vaccination.

New problems arose that drew him back to London. He was still in debt, and debtors in England at that time went to jail. Parliament had delayed paying his reward, and when it did pay, it imposed heavy taxes and fees. To make ends meet, he ceased vaccinating the poor, asking a friend to assume the responsibility. There then arose a problem with a Dr. Walker in the Royal Jennerian Society that Jenner felt obliged to resolve, and in which he unwisely became entangled.

Jenner was originally responsible for appointing Walker as the resident inoculator of the Royal Jennerian Society. Walker performed these duties at a place called Central House, where the poor received free vaccinations. He was a hostile, arrogant man. The slightest faults of patients irritated him. If a mother placed a child's clothing on his desk, he swept it onto the floor; if she happened to get in his way, he pushed her aside and made her stand childlike facing a corner of the room. If he could not hear how a mother spelled her name, he made her spell it loudly and slowly, ten times, in order to teach her a lesson; and if these incidents frightened her and she wanted to leave, he barricaded the exit—all the while making sarcastic remarks.

Walker also began charging some patients a fee. After much debate, the society agreed to allow him to continue this practice under certain circumstances. Then he committed what was, Jenner thought, an unpardonable sin: he wrote a letter to the editor of the *Medical and Physical Journal* in September 1804, describing a new method for obtaining some of the vaccine for other patients from a given patient's lesion. Jenner and many of his colleagues immediately claimed that this procedure impaired the effectiveness of vaccination. Much letter writing to the journal by various physicians and Walker ensued, debating the point. Jenner remained stubborn, unwilling to reach a compromise solution, a stubbornness that many regarded as the root cause of the disastrous events that followed. Jenner asked the society to dismiss Walker. Acrimonious debate ensued, dividing the members into those favoring and those against Walker. He eventually resigned on August 8, 1806.

Walker was determined to take his revenge. At first he refused to leave Central House, and when eventually he did, he took all patients' records with him. He rented a shop next door, enabling him to divert to his own practice patients who were on their way to Central House. Finally, on August 21, 1806, in direct competition with Central House, he opened the London Vaccine Institution with the lord mayor of London as its president.

The society replaced Walker with a twenty-two-year-old physician, James Sheridan Knowles, on October 2, 1806. Two years later Knowles was imprisoned for debt. This event was the straw that broke the camel's back; the Royal Jennerian Society closed its doors forever.

Now it was Jenner who was in danger of being imprisoned for debt. He turned to his old friends again, asking them to pressure Parliament into granting him another reward.

Parliament voted to ask the Royal College of Physicians of London to establish a Vaccination Committee, which in turn heard testimony from Jenner and others in favor of vaccination, as well as from those opposed to it. Parliament also asked the Royal College of Physicians of London to obtain the opinion of the Royal College of Physicians of Edinburgh and the Royal College of Physicians of Dublin, and the Colleges of Surgeons of Dublin, Edinburgh, and London. The Royal College in London also distributed questionnaires to its members, who strongly recommended vaccination. Feeling slighted at not being approached by Parliament directly, the College of Surgeons of London reported no conclusions. Jenner lamented the fact that a body of men so respected could let resentment of a slight affect their scientific judgment.

Meanwhile, word of Jenner's financial plight had reached the far corners of the earth. In India the citizens of Calcutta raised 4,000 pounds for him, Bombay sent 2,000 pounds, and the Presidency of Madras granted him 1,383 pounds. At long last, on July 29, 1807, the British Parliament voted a further grant of 20,000 pounds to Edward Jenner.

After the Royal Jennerian Society failed, Jenner advocated for government, rather than private individuals or organizations, to provide free vaccination. Through his political efforts, Parliament created the National Vaccine Establishment in 1809, naming him director and appointing a board of directors. Jenner intensely disliked some of the directors, particularly those whose views contradicted his own. After much political infighting, he resigned as director before the establishment held its first official meeting. The organization actually existed until 1867, at which time the Privy Council assumed the responsibilities.

Attacks on Jenner continued. Reports of failures of vaccination still poured in. Those opposed to vaccination taunted him with many articles, including a stinging satiric poem, and even a "Jenneric Opera," published in the *Medical Observer*. Much of his time turned to investigating the causes of vaccination failures and to answering the mounting, ever more stinging criticism.

Although this political activity had been consuming, Jenner found time to write a sixteen-page pamphlet, *Facts, for the Most Part Unobserved or Not Duly Noticed, Respecting Variolous Contagion*, in which he reported a series of patients who caught smallpox a second time. Neither prior natural smallpox nor variolation had protected these patients from a second attack. Modern physicians also have confirmed another observation first reported by Jenner, namely, that smallpox can infect a fetus without infecting the mother.

Now sixty years of age, Jenner in 1809 decided to "retire"—although he practiced medicine until 1822. He was appointed the local magistrate in Berkeley, and new hobbies interested him: gardening, farming, fossils, and geology. Always a scientist, but one whose mental abilities had begun to decline, he wrote a paper, "Observations on the Distemper in Dogs," in which he stated that he had vaccinated twenty dogs with cowpox all of which he (incorrectly) claimed had developed mild distemper. His eldest son, Edward Jr., developed tuberculosis and died on January 31, 1810. Jenner became deeply depressed, writing to a friend that he had no concept that the "gash would have been so deep."

Signs of a more serious mental problem made their appearance. Jenner began to experience the same auditory hallucinations and the same sudden jarring that had troubled him at age eight. He felt that his dejection rendered him unfit to perform his duties; and plays, concerts, and dancing had lost their appeal. To add to his woes, Catherine was now confined to bed, not only with tuberculosis but also with arthritis. She was, for all practical purposes, emotionally isolated from everyone, including Jenner himself.

On November 13, 1810, his sister Mary died, after falling down a flight of stairs. By now Jenner was experiencing not only depression and auditory hallucinations, but also agitation and "loss of courage." He worsened his condition by treating himself with brandy and opium.

At this point, Jenner's friend the Earl of Berkeley died. The House of Lords, which had begun hearings on his title and estate, summoned Jenner, the local magistrate, to testify. Jenner reported in a letter to Caleb Parry that every night after this experience he awoke, trembling, from a nightmare in which he dreamed that he had to appear before the Lord Chancellor, adding that such nerves as his were not worth owning.

At the beginning of August 1812, his second sister, Anne, developed a series of strokes from which she died on September 25. Jenner's spirits were at the lowest ebb he had ever experienced.

Why had this confident, outgoing, cheerful man become paranoid, depressed, and withdrawn? Did all these deaths and his own progressive illness remind him of his youth, when within two months he had become an orphan and faced the terrifying experience of variolation as it was then practiced? Did he fear being alone in the world in his old age; did he fear death itself; or did he have the earliest signs of a brain lesion?

To these questions there are no answers. He had other health problems as well: repeated attacks of abdominal pain, jaundice, and palpitations.

The College of Surgeons, now the Royal College of Surgeons, issued a circular stating that it would no longer variolate patients and would promote vaccination. This delighted Jenner, as did an honorary degree from Oxford. (True to his now-cantankerous personality, however, he at first refused to wear the cap and gown.) This honor made him desirous of another diploma denied him all his professional life, the Fellowship of the Royal College of Surgeons of London. But the Royal College proved less flexible than Oxford University; it demanded that he sit their examination and pass a test in Greek and Latin!

The event that pleased Jenner most was that his youngest son, Robert, was admitted to Oxford in 1815. During the boy's teenage years, Robert and his father had fought incessantly, his father at one point labeling him a drifter. Like his father before him, Robert had difficulty with Greek and Latin, but he had studied Hebrew in Cheltenham and excelled in it at Oxford. His proud father reported that he had acquired a good knowledge of what he described as "this wonderful language" in about three weeks. Also like his father, Robert enjoyed his avocations as much as his work; he managed to slip out for a vacation of grouse hunting in Scotland while the first term was still in progress. When his father discovered this indiscretion, his only comment was that it must be a great comfort to the grouse to find such a poor shot as Robert among them.

Jenner's brief period of happiness came to an abrupt end. On September 13, 1815, his wife died. Once again Jenner became deeply depressed. Despite vast differences in personality and in some of their opinions, he had loved Catherine and had accepted her religious views and her way of life.

After a time Jenner recovered sufficiently to see some patients, to serve again as the local magistrate, and to pursue his avocations. His interest in fine food revived somewhat; the local gentry revered his recipe for salted spareribs. Among his new interests was archaeology. He excavated some Roman ruins and was the first to discover the fossil of a sea-dwelling reptile in Britain. Writing medical articles still interested him, but their quality was now very poor and their conclusions rather ridiculous.

The caliber of his avocational writing, however, remained sterling almost to the end. Indeed, in 1820 at seventy-one years of age, Jenner submitted an article to the Royal Society concerning the migration of birds. This masterpiece of natural science appeared in the *Philosophical Transactions* a year after his death. In this article Jenner pointed out that the birds who visited England in the spring and summer and then disappeared did so because they migrated to a warmer climate. Previously it had been believed that those birds did not migrate but hibernated either under the ice of frozen ponds or beneath snow.

On August 5, 1820, Jenner had his first neurological seizure, after which he was unconscious for many hours. Although he finally regained consciousness and suffered no apparent paralysis, he realized that his life was drawing to a close. He who had always liked constant companionship now craved such associations even more. He often felt lonely, but was not visited often by either his daughter, Catherine, or by his surviving son, Robert.

Despite his ill health, Jenner at the end of 1821 visited his lifelong friend Caleb Parry in Bath. It would have been interesting to listen in on this final encounter of the two aged friends. One month after the visit Parry died; Jenner endured the freezing weather to attend his funeral.

On January 26, 1823, Jenner had another seizure and died. Surprisingly, although details of his forthcoming funeral were widely publicized in London, no Londoners came. It was a very small funeral at which all the attendees were local. Catherine and Robert of course were there, as were a few other relatives and a handful of other people. Among the mourners was one who felt the loss especially keenly: James Phipps, the first person ever to be vaccinated.

Orphaned at age five, a school dropout, and an indolent procrastinator, Edward Jenner rose by his own ability to become one of our greatest scientists. The world will forever owe him a debt of gratitude. He loved his vocation, medicine, in which he made two sensational discoveries: vaccination, and the fact that angina pectoris and heart attacks were caused by coronary artery disease and were aggravated by anger and irritation. Jenner also loved his avocations, and here he made equally remarkable discoveries. Ornithologists still claim that his work on the cuckoo and on bird migration ranks as outstanding in their field. Likewise, geologists maintain that his most impressive contribution to science was his discovery of the fossil remains of the prehistoric sea-dwelling reptile, the *Plesiosaurus.* What other scientist has achieved preeminence in fields as diverse as these?

Jenner's dream was that one day, because of his discovery, smallpox would cease to exist. That has happened in our century. He would be overwhelmed, were he alive today, to discover our employment of his methodology to inject dead bacteria or their toxins—as well as dead or weakened viruses—into the human body to develop resistance to scores of heretofore lethal diseases. Indeed, the wide range of diseases that vaccination can now combat might well have amazed him: bubonic plague, chicken pox, cholera, diphtheria, German measles, *Haemophilus influenzae* type B, hepatitis A, hepatitis B, influenza, measles, mumps, paratyphoid fever, pneumococcal pneumonia, poliomyelitis, rabies, Rocky Mountain spotted fever, tetanus, typhoid fever, typhus, whooping cough, and yellow fever. And perhaps in the not-too-distant future we may benefit from a vaccine that protects against AIDS.

5

Crawford Long and

Surgical Anesthesia

In 1591 Eufane MacAyane of Edinburgh, a young mother, was dragged from her home and taken away. Her pleas for mercy were ignored, and she was thrown into a pit and buried alive.[1]

What was her crime? She had just given birth to twin sons, and during her difficult labor she had asked for pain relief. The Church teachings of the day regarded the pain of childbirth as a punishment justly inflicted by God. Hoping to dissuade any woman from asking for relief from pain, presumably against God's wishes, the Church executed Eufane for this sin.

The concept that pain is a visitation from a just God dates at least from the earliest days of Christianity, but it may be even older.[2] Among Egyptian papyri from as much as forty-five hundred years ago are clear descriptions of what would have been painful surgical procedures. Although certain herbs were available then that could relieve pain, and were discussed in other papyri, the surgical descriptions themselves make no mention of them.

Similarly, the Babylonian Code of Hammurabi, which dates from about 2000 B.C., mentions surgery without relief of the accompanying pain. Indeed, before the modern era only a single surgeon in China, one surgeon in India, and a handful of Greek and Roman surgeons coupled the relief of pain with surgical procedures. By A.D. 150 to A.D. 200 a few Greek and Roman surgeons were giving herbs that not only relieved pain, but also put the patient to sleep, thereby approaching the capabilities of modern anesthetists. In fact, Dioscorides, a Greek army surgeon, was the first to use the term *anesthesia*.[3]

These isolated measures did not spread, in Christian Europe at least. In later centuries Muslim physicians did begin to use various herbs for the relief of pain, soaking a sponge in the appropriate herbs to be inhaled by the patient.[4] Known as soporific sponges, they were introduced in Christian Europe by monks between the fourteenth and seventeenth centuries. Contrary to their own teachings, the monks used such sponges on patients, but so many died anyway that their use was abandoned. Or they may have been discontinued because they were found to be ineffectual. (Recently a dozen of these ancient "soporific" recipes were collected by modern investigators and used to anesthetize experimental animals, but they were found to be useless.)

What was surgery like, then, without anesthesia?

When the first hospitals began to emerge in later centuries, they were often modeled after the London Hospital, built in 1791, which was designed with the operating room on the top floor. Outside the operating room was a bell; when an operation was contemplated, the bell was rung and all the nurses, physicians, and aides ran to the operating room and closed a heavy door so that the patient's screams could not be heard elsewhere. The entire hospital staff also helped to hold the patient down, gagging him or her if necessary.[5] The operating room featured a large skylight, so that natural daylight could compensate for the lack of electricity. The London Hospital, designed as it was in part because of the *lack* of anesthesia, became the model for hospital construction in all of Britain, Europe, and the United States.

Given the lack of anesthesia, a good surgeon was necessarily a fast surgeon. Speed was paramount; stopwatches timed the fastest. Napoleon's own surgeon, for example, could perform any amputation in less than one minute.

The first important advance in the development of anesthesia was the discovery in 1275, by the famous Spanish alchemist Raymundus Lullius, that if vitriol (sulfuric acid) was mixed with alcohol and distilled, a sweet, white fluid would result.[6] At first Lullius and his contemporaries called the fluid sweet vitriol; it was later called ether. Quite a future was in store for this simple chemical compound, even though six centuries would pass before its ultimate fate would be discovered.

In 1605 the famous alchemist Paracelsus, a Swiss physician, employed ether to relieve pain.[7] He was a medical, not a surgical, doctor, so he was not able to invent surgical anesthesia. After testing it on experimental animals, though, he administered ether to his medical patients who were in extreme pain. Amazingly, it would be the middle of the nineteenth century before anyone would again think to use ether for pain relief.

Another great advance was made by the English chemist Joseph Priestley, who discovered nitrous oxide, later called laughing gas, in 1772. Priestley did not recognize nitrous oxide as an anesthetic agent, but he did make a number of other enormously important discoveries, including the existence of oxygen and carbon monoxide.

However advanced his knowledge of science, Priestley committed two unpardonable sins in the England of his day. First, he was a liberal who supported the underclass in the French Revolution. Second, he was a Methodist minister who became a dissenting Unitarian minister, teaching that Jesus was a man, that God was all powerful, and that the principal benefits religion could bestow were compassion, appropriate morals, and high ethical standards. After upper-class mobs consisting of rich merchants and lords and ladies destroyed this dangerous radical's house, he fled to America in 1794, where he was given political and religious asylum.

After Priestley, the "pneumatic medicine" (medication by inhalation of various gases) he had helped to found became a kind of fad in England. One of its leading exponents was Thomas Beddoes, the physician and chemist from Berkeley, England, who was a neighbor of Jenner—whose vaccination process Beddoes had initially opposed and later strongly supported. Beddoes, a liberal like Priestley, was forced to leave his position as reader in chemistry at Oxford. In 1794 he traveled to Bristol, where he opened a Pneumatic Medicine Institution. Four years later he appointed Humphrey Davy, a brilliant twenty-two-year-old surgeon-chemist as superintendent.

Davy's youth was similar to Jenner's, in that he did very poorly at school, which he left at age thirteen. Without the qualifications to train as a physician, Davy apprenticed himself to a surgeon-apothecary. During his apprenticeship Davy developed an enormous interest in chemistry, which he essentially taught himself. It was he who introduced the term *laughing gas* for nitrous oxide, having inhaled it at the age of seventeen and feeling so exhilarated that he burst out laughing. Later he developed an inhaler for use with the gas.

In 1800 Davy published an astonishing book, the record of his research of the previous two years, in which he discussed in enormous detail the chemical, physical, and physiological properties of nitrous oxide.[8] The book was hailed as the work of a genius, particularly as its author was twenty-one at the time of publication and had been working on it for only two years.

In the book Davy recounted the eruption of a wisdom tooth. His entire gum became inflamed and painful, to the extent that he had to take nitrous oxide three times in one day, after which the pain in his jaw was temporarily relieved. He went so far as to suggest that nitrous oxide could be used for surgical operations, but Davy did not pursue this idea because he thought he had more meaningful work to do. That work included poetry; he was a poet of note, known and admired by the leading poets of his time. Samuel Taylor Coleridge remarked that if Davy had not been the greatest chemist of the age, he would have been the greatest poet. William Wordsworth asked Davy to edit the famous second edition of *Lyrical Ballads*, containing his own poems and *The Ancient Mariner* by Coleridge. Both Coleridge and Robert Southey took nitrous oxide for pleasure with Davy, prompting Southey to remark that the atmosphere of the highest conceivable heaven must certainly be nitrous oxide.

Davy left the Pneumatic Medicine Institution in 1801 to become a lecturer and later professor in chemistry at the Royal Institution in London. There he invented what he considered his most valuable contribution to science, the Davy lamp, which greatly reduced the risk of explosion in coal mines. Soon he became so famous that he was, for example, allowed to travel safely between London and Paris during the height of the Napoleonic Wars, to accept an award from the hands of Napoleon himself. Ever the prodigy, he was named Fellow of the Royal Society at age twenty-five, knighted at age thirty-two, and named president of the Royal Society at age forty-two, in which capacity he approved Jenner's work on bird migration for publication by the society, unfortunately after Jenner himself had died.

After Davy, the focus on nitrous oxide research moved to the United States, where William Barton wrote a medical thesis at the University of Pennsylvania in 1808, confirming Davy's observations about nitrous oxide.[9] Barton mentioned in his report that he had received a violent and very painful blow to the head, which nitrous oxide enabled him not to feel at all. Like Davy, he suggested using laughing gas as anesthesia during surgery. Again like Davy, he chose not to develop his idea further. Another thirty or so years would pass before the thought would be put to practical use.

When the concept of anesthesia was finally introduced, the people most interested were dentists and surgeons. Dentists needed only a very light anesthesia; surgeons needed, and still need, a deep anesthesia. Thus, there arose a division between dental and surgical anesthesia, and in discussions of the history of anesthesia it has, by common consent, become customary to focus on the history of surgical anesthesia.

Various American chemists realized after making anesthetics that inhaling them made people feel happy and gay. As a result, the chemists who made them organized "ether frolics" and "laughing-gas parties." As it happened, the first to use ether as a dental anesthetic was a chemistry student, William E. Clark, who had watched and participated in ether frolics himself. His dentist was Dr. Elija Pope. Clark suggested one day that Pope use it for dental extractions, no doubt figuring that a little frolic could only help with the pain. In January 1842 Pope's patient, a Miss Hovey, became the first person to have a tooth extracted painlessly, while under the influence of ether.

The initial use of anesthesia for surgical purposes was by Dr. Crawford Long. Born in Danville, Georgia, in 1815, Long was a graduate of Franklin College of Athens (Georgia) at the age of fourteen. He was a member of what must be the most distinguished graduating class in collegiate history, since every member would become famous. One became a governor, one a secretary of the treasury, two were senators, two Confederate generals, and (including Long himself) three became eminent scientists.

Long earned his medical degree at Transylvania University in Lexington, Kentucky, and at the University of Pennsylvania in Philadelphia, at the time the finest medical school in the country. He trained in surgery in New York City for eighteen months, then returned to Georgia in 1841 to establish a medical practice in Jefferson. The town was inhabited by only a few hundred souls, although Long's practice soon became larger than that, as he was an excellent doctor, kind and very devoted. His reputation spread. In fact, his practice grew to cover such a large geographic area that it could take him all day to go across Georgia's ravines and streams from one patient's home to another's. He was so busy and so dedicated that he was late to his own wedding, to Caroline Swain in 1842. He was with a very sick patient, and got to the wedding after nearly all the guests, thinking he must have changed his mind, had left. He had not; but after the ceremony he went back to his patient and did not see his bride for another day. Together they had twelve children, five of whom died of childhood illnesses.

Shortly after his wedding, several of the young men of Jefferson asked him to make some nitrous oxide for them, so that they could have laughing-gas parties. Long's response was that ether was just as good, and he promptly made some, which they all tried. The jollity was infectious, and ether frolics soon became fashionable in Jefferson and its environs.

At the jollifications he had helped to introduce, Long made an observation of profound importance. After a typical episode, he would be bruised from thrashing about under the influence of the ether, but could never remember feeling any pain when the actual bruises occurred. Long remembered these painless bumps when one of his patients, James N. Venable, had surgery scheduled several times for two cysts on his neck, but canceled each time because of the pain he feared he would have to undergo. Long invited him to some ether frolics to see that ether would not hurt him and was able in this way to convince Venable that ether was harmless. On March 30, 1842, Long poured some ether into a towel, let Venable inhale from it, and saw him become unconscious. Long removed one of the two cysts, without Venable's feeling any pain whatsoever. When Venable regained consciousness, he could not believe what had happened. Long had to show him the cyst to prove to Venable that it was gone. The experience was so successful that nine weeks later Long removed the second cyst, with the same happy result.

Long continued to give ether to his patients. In July 1842 he amputated a boy's toe painlessly, and by October 1846 he had administered surgical anesthesia successfully to eight patients. On each occasion there were numerous witnesses who confirmed what had happened, a fact that would be meaningful in what was to come. In addition, Long was the first to use anesthesia for an obstetrical procedure, in December 1845. So by the time he was twenty-six, he had become the first person in the long history of medicine to use surgical anesthesia and, by the time he was twenty-nine, the first person to use obstetrical anesthesia.

Long moved to Atlanta in 1850 and a year later to Athens, Georgia. During the Civil War news reached Athens that a division of federal cavalry was approaching, with orders to burn the city. Long reached home just as his daughter Frances and her younger brother were fleeing. He gave Frances a glass jar containing a roll of papers on which he had recorded evidence of his discovery of surgical anesthesia. Frances buried the jar in a wooded area, from which it was recovered after the war.

Long practiced surgery and anesthesia until June 16, 1878, when he died suddenly from a massive cerebral hemorrhage while delivering a baby to the local congressman's wife. His dying words were, "Care for the mother and child first."

Dr. Long certainly was the first person to employ ether to abolish both consciousness and pain in patients undergoing surgery. But he did not publish this stunning achievement until 1849, seven years after his discovery.[10] Moreover, were it not for the competing claims of two dentists and one physician in 1846, it is doubtful that Long would ever have published his article.

It is now time to describe the three other claims. Before doing so, however, we should mention that the physician, Charles Jackson, and probably one of the dentists, William Thomas Green Morton, had visited the tiny village of Jefferson in the spring of 1842, at the precise time that Dr. Long had given ether to his first patient.[11] It is almost inconceivable that this earthshaking event did not serve as a focus of admiring discussion among the four hundred citizens of Jefferson. It is also almost inconceivable that

Dr. Jackson and the dentist were not immediately apprised by the villagers of the ether discovery.

We emphasize this visit because Jackson, on returning to Harvard University after his visit to Jefferson, claimed he had suffered a sore throat of such intensity that he had given himself some ether, which rendered him unconscious as he sat in his chair. He claimed that this strange medical episode had taken place in February 1842, conveniently a month earlier than Long's first anesthetic procedure. His chair is still part of the anesthesia exhibit at Massachusetts General Hospital in Boston. Many who were aware of Jackson's personality and previous claims, however, doubted the validity of his new discovery.

Jackson was born in Plymouth, Massachusetts, in 1805 and received his M.D. with honors from Harvard in 1829. He was on the medical faculty there and at Massachusetts General Hospital, and had an encyclopedic knowledge. He worked hard, publishing more than four hundred papers, and all the evidence is that Harvard was proud of him.

Although he was undoubtedly brilliant, he also had sociopathic tendencies. His colleagues remembered him as being overcompetitive, deceitful, sly, manipulative, and highly suspicious. At different times in his career he falsely claimed a number of discoveries that had been made by other persons—which, curiously, did not seem to have bothered Harvard. In any event, he was never disciplined for these indiscretions.

One colleague, for example, William Beaumont, was world famous for his studies on digestion. He had an unusual patient named Alexis St. Martin, an islander put in Beaumont's custody by Congress and by the surgeon general himself. St. Martin had a gunshot wound to the stomach that had remained permanently open, so Beaumont had only to look inside to see the digestive processes at work.

Eventually Beaumont sent Jackson a sample of St. Martin's gastric juices for chemical analysis. Jackson realized at once that if he could study St. Martin himself, he would become world famous. He tried to hide the islander from Beaumont and, without telling Beaumont, circulated a petition in Congress in 1834, asking that Alexis St. Martin be put in Jackson's care. The surgeon general, hearing this, was enraged and Jackson's petition failed.[12]

Again, in 1832, Jackson met Samuel Morse, a fellow passenger on a ship returning from Europe. One afternoon a group sat in the lounge discussing electromagnetism, and someone asked Jackson about the relationship between the flow of electricity and the length of a wire. Jackson answered the question, and Morse commented that it might be possible to transmit messages in this way. When he reached the United States, Morse went on to invent the telegraph, which he patented in 1837. But Jackson claimed that *he* had invented the telegraph. The case went all the way to the Supreme Court, which subsequently ruled that Morse was indeed the inventor and that Jackson had played no role whatsoever.

On yet another occasion, Jackson claimed that he, not Schonbein, had invented gun cotton. Jackson would make other claims too, as the reader will discover.

It is appropriate now that we describe the role of Horace Wells in the discovery of anesthesia. Wells was born in Hartford, Vermont, in 1815 and graduated from Harvard Dental School in 1834. He taught there for many years, was very learned, and wrote articles in the dental journals of the day.

Wells, however gifted, was an unstable man.[13] He intermittently gave up his practice, once going to France to buy art, which he sold for a profit in the United States, and on another occasion leaving to manufacture portable baths and stoves. He was highly religious and once considered entering the ministry. Overexuberant at times, he still was easily depressed, and the opinions of others unduly swayed him.

On December 10, 1844, Wells attended a nitrous oxide party given by Dr. Gardner Q. Colton. He sat next to someone inhaling the laughing gas, who severely bruised his leg but who felt no pain. Wells immediately recognized that laughing gas might work as a dental anesthetic. He himself had a badly decayed tooth, so the next day he asked Colton to give him laughing gas while a colleague removed the tooth. As he did so, Wells felt no pain. When he had recovered from the anesthesia, he called out excitedly that this was the greatest discovery in the history of the world.

Before we continue Wells's story, it is opportune at this time to introduce the second dentist, William Thomas Green Morton, in our account of the discovery of surgical anesthesia.

Morton probably was the mysterious dentist who visited Jefferson in 1842. He had been taught dentistry at Harvard by Wells, who later took him as a partner in his private dental practice. In 1844, however, Morton decided to study medicine at Harvard and had Jackson as his preceptor. This strange union of distinctly sociopathic personalities resulted in so many conflicts and such confusion that even the U.S. Congress was baffled.

Morton, hearing of Wells's discovery of the anesthetic power of nitrous oxide, became tremendously enthusiastic about it. A medical student at Harvard, he arranged for Wells to demonstrate his discovery before a surgical, not a dental, class of students. Dr. John C. Warren, the world-famous physician then at Harvard, speedily approved the demonstration.

This historic demonstration was scheduled for the surgical amphitheater at the Massachusetts General Hospital in Boston in January 1845. Wells's fragile ego, though, was about to receive an unexpected blow. The apparatus he used to administer the laughing gas involved a wooden mouthpiece and a stopcock attached to a 2-liter bag of oiled silk. This was not large enough to anesthetize the patient; he needed at least 30 liters—but that, of course, he did not know.[14] Another problem was that his patient was a terrified boy with a bad tooth. Wells was only able to administer a partial anesthesia, the boy screamed, and—instead of the applause he expected—he heard hisses and boos and was bodily thrown out of the amphitheater. Wells was devastated, although the boy said when he recovered that he could not remember any pain. The medical students who had seen the demonstration remained unimpressed, and Wells went into a deep depression.

He recovered, however, and within a short period used laughing gas to anesthetize forty patients during his dental procedures. All of these patients furnished him with written affidavits declaring that they felt no pain, and witnesses were present at each procedure. Still, no one at the hospital believed his story.

Morton, shortly prior to Wells's debacle before the Harvard surgeons and medical students, began to associate with Jackson as well as with Wells. Jackson, unaware of the probable fact that Morton, like himself, had visited Jefferson and had become quite familiar with the anesthetic power of ether, confided to Morton that ether was an outstanding anesthetic. Morton's immediate response was "Ether? What is it?"

Morton later claimed under oath that when Jackson told him about ether, he already had been experimenting with it but had hidden this activity from Jackson. He later insisted that he had anesthetized a fish, some insects, and a puppy, as well as himself; but one of his fellow medical students later told the U.S. Congress that Morton had never done any experiments at all.

Apparently Morton did try to anesthetize two dental students with ether; but both became agitated, not anesthetized. At this point Morton realized that he would have to join up with Jackson, who he knew possessed genuine knowledge. Jackson pointed out that Morton had used impure commercially made ether, and that for anesthetic purposes they would have to make the ether themselves. This they did and decided that they could make a lot of money through the strategic employment of secrecy. Jackson had the idea of mixing ether with aromatic oils, to disguise its true nature; he and Morton patented it as Letheon and tried to keep its contents secret.[15]

Morton used this new product on Eben Frost on September 30, 1846. Jackson told Morton exactly how to administer the anesthesia and was convinced that it would work—and it did. Morton extracted the patient's tooth painlessly; witnesses were present; and the *Boston Journal* heralded the new discovery in an article published the very next day.

Morton now approached John Warren about a test. His request was similar to the one he had made on Wells's behalf two years before. Again Warren said yes, and his house surgeon, Dr. C. F. Heywood, wrote Morton proposing that at 10 A.M. on Friday morning, October 16, 1846, surgical anesthesia be given to a patient having a tumor of the jaw removed. A young surgeon, Dr. Henry Jacob Bigelow, arranged the details of the demonstration, inviting all of Boston's leading surgeons (but, oddly, no medical students).

Morton did not appear. An alarmed Bigelow went to Morton's office, where he found an equally alarmed Morton packing his bags to leave town. Bigelow managed to persuade him to go ahead. Letheon, after all, he encouraged Morton, could be effective. Bigelow and Morton arrived at the surgical amphitheater at Massachusetts General Hospital just as Warren was about to make his incision. Morton made up an excuse on the spot (something about waiting for his instrument maker to complete a new inhaler). He then administered the Letheon.

Unlike Long, who had poured his ether onto a towel, Morton used an inhaler. What he feared would happen did not happen—or only partially happened—because, like Wells, he had problems with his inhaler. In Morton's case, the inhaler had a wooden spigot but no valve. During the incision the patient felt no pain, but later began to speak incoherently and became agitated. Afterward the patient said that he had felt as though his neck were being scratched, and he was apparently aware that an operation was proceeding.

This time there were no boos or hisses. The visiting surgeons and Warren himself were stunned by the favorable outcome. At the next operation Morton anesthetized a patient for Dr. Heywood, again using Letheon. The patient was having a large tumor removed from his left arm and, thanks to Morton's improved inhaler with brass inspiratory and expiratory valves (still on exhibit at the Massachusetts General Hospital), the anesthesia worked very well. The patient was unconscious throughout, could remember no pain, and groaned only occasionally toward the end of the procedure.[16]

After this second, highly successful anesthesia, Warren, Heywood, and Bigelow learned that Morton and Jackson had patented Letheon. They said publicly that this was unethical. When Jackson heard their statement, he withdrew his name from the patent but entered into a written agreement with Morton according to which Morton would pay him $500 and 10 percent of all future profits from the use of Letheon.

When Dr. Warren learned of these machinations, he prohibited the use of Letheon and banned Morton and his new anesthesia from the Commonwealth of Massachusetts. Morton was therefore forced to reveal that Letheon was just ether, since without some degree of medical cooperation he would never be able to work as an anesthetist again. Warren asked Morton why he had tried to conceal the ether with aromatic oils. Morton lied, replying that the oils made a more powerful anesthetic. These claims notwithstanding, he and Jackson later canceled their patent application.

On November 9, 1846, Bigelow delivered a lecture before the Boston Society of Medical Improvement on the new anesthesia, and on November 18 published reports of Morton's two successful cases in the *Boston Medical and Surgical Journal*.[17]

Within days of the publication of Bigelow's article, worldwide attention was being paid to the new anesthesia. In the glow of all this publicity, Jackson, Morton, and Wells each claimed to have discovered it. The other claimants to the throne — William E. Clark, who had given the first dental anesthesia, and Crawford Long — at this point were silent. Clark wanted no part of all the publicity, and Long could not be bothered either — and would not have been, except for the efforts of his home state senator.

Shortly thereafter Jackson and Morton signed an agreement, with the help of advisers and lawyers, claiming to be codiscoverers of surgical anesthesia. Wells learned of the agreement and felt it was a slap in the face. It may have been a contributing factor in his taking his own life in 1848 by opening a vein in his arm and inhaling ether as he did so.

The strange story of the discovery of surgical anesthesia continued to become stranger. Within days of signing the agreement with Morton, Jackson, ever the deceitful schemer, wrote to the French Academy of Sciences and stated that he was the sole discoverer of surgical anesthesia. When Morton heard of the claim, he went back to his lawyers and advisers, broke off the agreement, and thereafter claimed that he had been the sole discoverer.

This bickering between Jackson, Morton, and for a short while Wells about who first discovered surgical anesthesia became so bitter that the U.S. Congress in 1847 stepped in to decide who indeed was the first discoverer. This matter, eventually called the Ether Controversy, preoccupied Congress for sixteen years, despite the onset of the Civil War.

Morton's claims were supported by two powerful friends. The first was Daniel Webster, the best-known orator and lawyer of his time, founder of the Whig Party, and a vastly influential United States senator. The second was Oliver Wendell Holmes, professor of anatomy at Harvard, already famous as an essayist, novelist, and poet. Despite all this firepower on Morton's behalf, Congress decided that Morton definitely did not discover surgical anesthesia. Many witnesses substantiated the fact that he had learned everything he knew about ether from Jackson, and they also testified that they had heard Morton assert frequently that Jackson had, in fact, invented the anesthesia.

William Morton came to be called the Great Pretender in congressional reports, because of his initial "pretending" to Jackson that he knew nothing about ether. He went on to limit his practice to anesthesia, but shortly after the notable developments of 1846, he underwent severe financial and emotional problems. In 1868, at age forty-nine, he died a relatively young man for reasons that remain obscure.

Congress also decided that Wells had definitely not invented surgical anesthesia, because he attempted only dental anesthesia. In any case he had by then committed suicide and was no longer available to claim the prize.

The contest, therefore, was between Jackson and Long, at least as Congress had come to see it. Given the powerful advocates on both sides of the question, Congress was unable to decide on the identity of the discoverer of surgical anesthesia. Incredibly, it asked the coclaimants to resolve the question themselves! They ordered Jackson to visit Long in Georgia, which he did. As was his wont, Long was courtly, pleasant, and deferential to the older man, but the two were unable to settle the dispute. Shortly after leaving Georgia, Jackson became demented and remained so for the rest of his life.

Thus, Long was the only claimant to lead a normal life after 1846; the others died either harassed or insane. Long remained calm in response to the tumult and continued to treat the whole affair as if it were of little consequence.

Various learned dental and medical societies also debated the question and in the end were as divided as Congress had been. Each society established a position that continues in force to this day. In 1864, for example, the American Dental Association, and in 1870 and again in 1872 the American Medical Association, passed resolutions to the effect that Wells had discovered anesthesia. That the American Medical Association would make this contention is interesting, since Wells by his own admission had never performed any surgical anesthesia. Still, he had demonstrated his dental anesthetic techniques before the "surgical" class at Harvard, which may account for the position taken by the medical group.

In 1913 the electors of the New York University Hall of Fame also debated the issue at great length. It was pointed out that Long was in a tiny, very isolated village of some four hundred individuals, that all his witnesses were members of the general public and possessed no medical training; nor were there local medical societies to which he could present a paper, since he was the only doctor for miles around. In the Georgia countryside information traveled slowly and Long had, for his own reasons, delayed publishing his results until 1849. It is conceivable, but unlikely, that Long did not fully realize the significance of his work.

Morton, on the other hand, had worked at one of the most famous universities, and his first patient was referred by the best-known surgeon in the world. His witnesses were other surgeons in the Boston area, and his results were reported almost immediately. The news would spread: indeed, by mid-1847 nearly all large hospitals in Britain, Europe, Cuba, South America, and South Africa were routinely using ether as a surgical anesthetic, based on Bigelow's article reporting Morton's two cases.

In the debate at New York University, the most famous participant was Sir William Osler, who convinced the electors to name Morton the discoverer. His argument was that, in science, credit should go to the man who convinces the world, not to the man who first has the idea or who proves that it works. A curious argument, but one the electors accepted, naming Morton the discoverer of surgical anesthesia. We wonder whether, if Osler had known that Morton visited Jefferson in 1842, he still would have insisted that Morton be judged the discoverer.

The American College of Surgeons, meeting in Atlanta in 1921, named Long the discoverer and created the Crawford Long Association, which in 1926 erected a statue of Long in Statutory Hall in Washington, D.C. Later a hospital in Atlanta was named the Long Memorial Hospital in his honor, and since that time most surgeons throughout the world have accepted Crawford Long as the discoverer of surgical anesthesia. We too have decided to award the honor to this backwoods surgeon.

The next major development in the history of surgical anesthesia occurred in Britain, where John Snow, a twenty-three-year-old London general practitioner, became the first full-time physician-anesthetist in the world. (Morton, the reader will recall, also practiced anesthesia full-time but never got his medical degree and remained a dentist all his life.)

Snow was very scientifically inclined and improved the ether inhalers so that the anesthetist could determine and control the ether-air mixture being given the patient. He was the first to analyze the physiological effects of anesthetics, publishing his results in a famous monograph on the subject.[18]

Later, Sir James Simpson, professor of obstetrics at the University of

Edinburgh, began to advocate the use of anesthesia for obstetrics. It was brave of him, and of his first patient, to do so in view of what had happened to Eufane MacAyane in the same city some three centuries earlier. As he feared, the Calvinist Church in Edinburgh opposed the use of anesthesia for obstetrics, saying that the Holy Bible itself maintained that women must bear children in pain. Fortunately, the Church did not bury him or his patient alive, perhaps because he had a powerful advocate in Queen Victoria, whose obstetrician he had become. He was also able to defend himself, quoting the circumstances attending the birth of Eve as described in Genesis 2:21: "And the Lord God caused a deep sleep to fall upon Adam, and he slept; and he took one of his ribs, and closed up the flesh . . . thereof."

As it developed, ether, the first anesthetic, had many disadvantages. Among other things, it caused vomiting and bronchial irritation. The search therefore was on to make a better, safer, less toxic anesthetic.

In 1831 the American chemist Samuel Guthrie was the first to make chloroform. He did not recognize it as an anesthetic, even though his eight-year-old daughter tasted some of the new chemical (he having left the room) and became unconscious for several hours despite his very physical attempts to awaken her.[19]

Some years later Simpson, the obstetrician in Edinburgh, asked a chemist friend whether he could recommend a better anesthetic than ether. The friend had heard of Guthrie's daughter and thought this new substance, chloroform, might do the trick.

Simpson first anesthetized himself and found the results positive, with no adverse side effects. He therefore gave chloroform to his niece during the delivery of her child. Soon thereafter he was called to deliver Queen Victoria's eighth child, Prince Leopold, on April 7, 1853. He called in his friend John Snow, and asked him to give the queen a chloroform anesthetic. Snow poured a small amount into the queen's handkerchief and held it under her nose. It was a huge success! The queen remained conscious but felt no pain, and the very next day newspapers trumpeted around the world the story of her exposure to the new anesthetic. From that day forward the Calvinists of Edinburgh remained silent.

Chloroform soon became the anesthetic of choice of all physicians practicing in Britain and Germany. Unfortunately, as with ether, it turned out that there were problems. Slowly it was learned that chloroform could cause liver damage, and that five times more patients died after having been given chloroform than after ether. Leading physicians in Britain and Germany suggested limiting its use.

While the controversy concerning the possible toxicity of chloroform raged, a truly momentous advance in surgical anesthesia occurred in 1880. The renowned British surgeon Sir William Macewan passed a metal tube into the mouth of a patient, pushed it down the throat, past the vocal cords, to enter the trachea. Thus was born endotracheal anesthesia. Without it, the many cardiac and pulmonary operations performed today would be impossible.[20] For endotracheal anesthesia permits the contemporary anesthetist to inflate and deflate the lungs, which otherwise would lay collapsed by the entrance of atmospheric air as soon as the chest was opened.

Although the German surgeon Frederich Trendelenburg had designed and employed a metal tube with an inflatable cuff a decade earlier, he could only use his tube by incising a hole in the trachea—not a pleasant wound preliminary to the major surgical wound to be sustained by the patient.

Macewan's tracheal tube was rigid, which made it difficult to insert and capable of damaging the tissues. Franz Kuhn of Kessel, Germany, developed a metal tube flexible enough to be inserted through the nose if necessary; shortly thereafter, Dorrance and Janeway put Trendelenburg-style balloons around flexible silastic tube, which they inflated, preventing aspiration into the lungs and rendering the administration of anesthesia easier still.[21]

With the rapid development of these new intubation methods, physicans found that it was easier to insert the tube if the patient was given a light anesthesia first. But in 1919 the British anesthetist Sir Ivan Magill developed what turned out to be an amazing technique: first anesthetizing the patient's throat with cocaine, then placing two tubes—one through the nose and one through the mouth—into the windpipe of the fully conscious patient without using any of the newly available sophisticated instruments for entering the trachea. Magill and his elaborate new technique rapidly became world famous, and other anesthetists came from everywhere to learn from him. But Magill, intent on remaining the only anesthetist in the world capable of inserting tubes into the windpipe via the nose and mouth, kept secret the fact that he anesthetized the throat with cocaine prior to the insertion of the tubes.

While inserting these various tubes as an aid to anesthesia was becoming standard practice in the United Kingdom and in Europe, the United States on the whole remained fixed on simpler, less effective methods. This fact upset Arthur Gudell, an anesthetist, who realized that he would have to come up with something dramatic to get his conservative colleagues to consider the merits of the fancy new endotracheal tubes.

So in 1926 he went around the country with what became his famous Dunking Dog Shows, in which he anesthetized and intubated his pet dog, Airway. He immersed Airway in an aquarium, in front of an audience of anesthetists. He discontinued the anesthesia, pulled Airway out of the water, removed the tube, and allowed Airway to awaken perfectly safely—after which Airway, faithful to the end, would bounce up, shake water on the conservative audience, and stalk out of the room. Everyone expected, of course, that Airway would drown. Gudell was demonstrating the virtues of the inflatable cuff, which would seal Airway's windpipe and allow him to breathe as through a snorkel. Very shortly after these extravaganzas, endotracheal anesthesia became common practice in the United States.[22]

In 1932 Ralph Waters, at the University of Wisconsin in Madison, accidentally inserted a tube down the full length of a patient's windpipe, into the right bronchial tube itself, where, again accidentally, he inflated the cuff. At first the mistake irritated him; but in a flash he realized that a longer tube, like the one he was using, inflated in the way he had inflated it, could be used to ventilate one lung while the surgeon was operating on the other. With this accidental discovery, lung surgery became possible, and another era dawned.[23]

As more practical methods of administering anesthetics were being developed, new anesthetic gases were discovered, particularly after World War I. Trilene in 1917 was followed by ethylene in 1923 and divinyl ether in 1931. These were succeeded by cyclopropane and halohane.

Cyclopropane was the anesthetic of choice in the 1930s and 1940s, since it was potent at low concentrations, and particularly because it suppressed breathing.[24] The anesthetist thus could use the air bag to regulate and control the patient's breathing, which was a major advance in anesthesiology.

The next step forward was the introduction of halothane in 1956; this substance was not only safe and potent, but nonflammable.[25] Until then nearly all surgical anesthetics were flammable. Since surgeons by this time were using electric currents for electrocautery, fires and even explosions occasionally resulted. Halothane rendered this bizarre possibility a thing of the past.

The next big advance involved the development of curare, not an anesthetic but a substance that paralyzed the voluntary muscles. (All muscles are either voluntary or involuntary: voluntary muscles include the arms, the legs, and the mouth; involuntary muscles work without conscious control and include, for example, the heart.)

For many centuries it was known that South American Indians poisoned the tips of their hunting arrows with juices from various poisonous plants in the rain forests. The advantage was that merely by hitting the animal anywhere on its body, it would be paralyzed from the effects of the poison. News of this remarkable substance reached Europe extraordinarily fast. In 1516, within a generation of Columbus' discovery of the New World, Peter Martyr de Anghera had described seeing curare in action.[26] But it was 170 years before G. Maggravius would coin the term *curare*.

More years would pass before anyone thought to use curare for purposes other than hunting. Its potential usefulness as a muscle relaxant during anesthesia was hindered by the fact that clinically pure curare was not available until 1935, but in 1942 it began to be used on a large scale.[27] It relaxed the patient's muscles, making the surgeon's (especially the abdominal surgeon's) work much easier, since otherwise the great muscles would clench. It also enabled the anesthetist to control the patient's breathing. By 1948 some eight thousand patients had received curare. Many more would have, had enough curare been available. To satisfy the demand, a synthetic version was finally produced in 1949.

Emil Fischer, in Berlin in 1903, was the first to develop a number of barbiturates that could be injected.[28] The safest, Pentothal, was developed in 1935 and was used to put the patient rapidly into a very pleasant sleep so that inhalation anesthetics could be used subsequently.[29] Many other safe, injectable anesthetics have since been developed, and they currently enjoy wide clinical use.

In addition to general anesthetics, the need for local anesthetics was evident early on. Although complications of general anesthesia are relatively rare, they do occur. Moreover, there are many times when a general anesthetic is not necessary, including the majority of trips to the dentist.

Then too, after a general anesthetic most people need several hours to recover. The goal was to find a way to numb the nerve supply to one area of the body only.

The use of local anesthesia has an ancient history. For centuries the Indians in Peru used small circular saws to cut holes in people's heads—to remove evil spirits or sometimes to remove objects that had penetrated the brain. The person doing the procedure would chew the leaves of the coca plant, then drip his saliva on the patient's wound to anesthetize it.

Scherzer was the first modern investigator to chew coca, and he noticed that it made his tongue numb.[30] Albert Nieman, a German, was the first to obtain a chemically pure cocaine and to give it its name.

Carl Koller, an eye physician, first used cocaine to anesthetize the eyes of frogs. He reported his results to an eye congress in Heidelberg on September 15, 1884, after which its use as a local anesthetic became widespread—first in the eye, then in the mouth, nose, and throat, and finally in the urethra.

It was the pioneering work of America's most famous surgeon, William S. Halsted of Johns Hopkins Hospital, that was chiefly responsible for the general employment of cocaine for local anesthesia by its injection into nerves supplying the area to be surgically treated. This prestigious surgeon not only injected cocaine into the nerves of hundreds of patients undergoing minor surgical procedures, but also repeatedly injected his own nerves in experimental studies. Further, Halsted introduced the use of rubber gloves in surgery, initially not to protect the surgical patient but to protect the hands of his wife, who as a nurse assisted him in the operating room. After injecting over one thousand patients, Halsted published his classic paper announcing cocaine's marvelous anesthetic capability.[31]

What Halsted did not announce in any medical journal was his intractable, lifelong addiction to cocaine, which intermittently played havoc with his surgical career. He carefully concealed his addiction and only revealed it, toward the end of his life, to his close friend Sir William Osler.

Following the success of cocaine, interest switched to the possibility of numbing the big nerves emerging from the spinal cord, which would permit anesthetization of a much larger area. Around the spinal cord itself is a layer of spinal fluid, contained in a membrane, which is in turn surrounded by an outer tube. This tube is separated from the walls of a bony canal (formed by the vertebrae) by a fat-filled space called the epidural space. In 1888 Leonard Corning of New York tried injecting cocaine into the epidural space and was very successful.[32] His procedure is now called epidural anesthesia. In 1899 August Bier, a German, injected cocaine directly into the spinal fluid, calling his procedure spinal anesthesia.[33]

The next significant advance occurred in Germany in 1897 via Heinrich Braun, who added epinephrine to the cocaine solution. The epinephrine causes the muscles of the very small arteries to contract, reducing the blood supply to the area in question. This process decreases the amount of local anesthetic that is absorbed, which means that it is less toxic generally, yet its effects will last longer in the area in which it is injected.

Fortunately, cocaine is no longer used for anesthetic purposes. It has been completely replaced by novocaine, which was synthesized in 1899 by the German chemist Alfred Eihorn and first employed for anesthetic purposes by Braun in 1905.[34]

Such in brief is the history of the discovery of anesthesia. It may appear fantastic to the casual reader that five full centuries had to elapse from the time ether was first made by an alchemist before this simple substance was determined by Crawford Long, surgeon in a minuscule village, to keep people asleep no matter how deeply their tissues and organs were ravaged by surgeons.

The same casual reader might be more astonished to learn that even seven centuries after this simple alcohol and sulfuric acid substance was discovered, medical scientists—despite huge amounts of research effort—still have not been able to find the answer to the most fundamental question of all: how does the administration of ether lead to unconsciousness and lack of awareness of any sort of pain? Before the twenty-first century has ended, however, it is likely that medicine will have found the elusive answer.

6

Wilhelm Roentgen and

the X-ray Beam

A cadet entering the United States Military Academy at West Point pledges neither to lie, cheat, or steal, nor to tolerate any other cadet who has committed such a misdemeanor or felony. In 1862, a naive seventeen-year-old rather phlegmatic Prussian lad, who was not a military cadet but a simple student, was pressed by the headmaster of his gymnasium to reveal the identity of a classmate guilty of drawing an unflattering portrait of one of the school's teachers. He refused to do so. He refused, even though he was aware that the headmaster knew he had recognized the culprit. He simply would not betray his classmate. Not only was he expelled because of his recalcitrance, but he could not subsequently be admitted into any other Dutch or German gymnasium. Thus he could never receive an *abitur* (a diploma) certifying that he had graduated from a gymnasium. And without an abitur, admission to any university as a regular student was impossible.[1]

Actually, this handicap may have been responsible for his later discovery of the X ray. Unable to enter any university in Germany or Holland because he lacked a gymnasium diploma, William Conrad Roentgen was forced to matriculate in 1865 at the Polytechnical School in Zurich, which did not require the abitur. In three years there he did not take any courses in theoretical or general physics, but only mechanical engineering subjects in which he learned to construct intricate apparatuses of all kinds. It was his marvelous skill in designing and constructing instruments that attracted the attention of Dr. August Kundt, one of the most distinguished theoretical physicists in Europe. Kundt, brilliant at conjuring up new theories and laws of physics, recognized that the young Roentgen, although relatively lackluster in his engineering courses, did know how to transform, with almost fantastic subtlety, glass, metal, and rubber into exquisite instruments—instruments that detected and measured physical phenomena that confirmed some of Kundt's theoretical concepts.

He persuaded the young Roentgen to forget about becoming a mechanical engineer, despite his having just obtained a degree in that field. He urged Roentgen to become his assistant at the University of Zurich. He also made it possible for Roentgen simultaneously to study for a doctorate in theoretical physics, despite the academic stain of his failure to obtain a gymnasium diploma.

When Kundt left the University of Zurich in 1870 for a new position at the University of Würzburg, and again when in 1872 he accepted a post at the University of Strasbourg, Roentgen faithfully followed, always working as Kundt's assistant. Finally in 1874, at the age of twenty-nine, he overcame the barrier of the missing abitur. He was appointed an instructor at the University of Strasbourg and in 1876 was made an assistant professor. Three years later he parted from Kundt, accepting a full professorship at the University of Giessen.

Let us return to the year 1872. Roentgen, aged twenty-seven and firmly established as an assistant to Kundt at the University of Würzburg, decided to marry Bertha Ludwig, the daughter of a prosperous, very well educated innkeeper. Bertha was slender, reasonably attractive, fairly well educated, and totally satisfied to be the wife of a physics professor. She was six years older than Roentgen and subject to intermittent but prolonged bouts of psychosomatic illness. Neither of these factors ever seemed to interfere with a marriage that continued until she died at eighty years of age. Indeed, the need for Roentgen to give her multiple injections of morphine daily during the last few years of her life did not appear to be annoying or burdensome to him, and he seemed unaware of the probability that she had become addicted to the drug.

The Roentgens lived a happy, essentially eventless life during their nine years at Giessen. Her psychosomatic illnesses isolated Roentgen from a busy (but to him fruitless) social life. Bertha always seemed to recover well enough to accompany him on their annual holiday in Switzerland. After four childless years they adopted Bertha's six-year-old niece, also named Bertha. In 1888 Roentgen rather regretfully left Giessen to accept a professorship of theoretical physics at the prestigious University of Würzburg.

From the attainment of his doctorate in 1869 to his departure in 1888, Roentgen lived very comfortably in a house ably cared for by Bertha and a staff composed of a housekeeper, a cook, and a maid. Although he was a poor lecturer and not particularly liked by students because of his aloofness and stern insistence on stellar performance, he managed to perform creditable laboratory experiments. He meticulously measured the physical alterations that occurred in various substances when subjected to barometric, light, and electrical changes. He learned that when a dielectric material (for example, a piece of glass) is moved between two electrically charged condenser plates, a current arises from the dielectric substance. With the possible exception of that early work, it is doubtful that Roentgen would be remembered today for any of his research prior to his magnificent discovery of the X ray.

Among Roentgen's important predecessors was Sir William Crookes, England's most distinguished physicist.[2] Having discovered thallium in 1861, he became interested in investigating the possible effects of discharges of electricity on rare gases. To accomplish this sort of research, he had to create an atmosphere containing only the specific gas he wished to study. He constructed what is now called a Crookes tube, at first fabricated as a glass cylinder whose air had been evacuated by means of a pump, thus creating a vacuum. The cylinder also contained electrodes for the discharge of an electric current produced by an induction coil–battery setup. He wanted to observe the changes that might occur in various rare gases and other substances when he exposed them to a high-voltage current passing from the cathode to the anode, both sealed in his vacuum cylinder. The passage of the current was effected by the emission of what came to be known as cathode rays.

It happened that Crookes occasionally dropped wooden cassettes containing unexposed photographic plates onto the same table upon which he had stationed his vacuum cylinder. Some time later, when he had occasion to use these plates, he found that some of them were flawed by shadows. It never occurred to him that the plates, seemingly protected from light by the wooden cassettes, still might have been exposed to a new type of ray generated by the cathode rays. He wrote to the manufacturer, complaining that the photographic plates had been light damaged.[3]

Similarly it never occurred to the distinguished physicist Phillip Lenard to investigate why slips of paper covered with barium platinocyanide salts and lying near his Crookes tube began to fluoresce as soon as he produced cathode rays by running a current through the cylinder. After Roentgen had discovered the X ray, Lenard in his 1905 Nobel Prize lecture lamely said, "In reality I had made several unexplainable observations which I carefully kept for future investigations, unfortunately not started in time, which must have been the effects of traces of wave radiation."

Even in this Nobel lecture, delivered ten years after Roentgen's discovery of the X ray and its worldwide acceptance, Lenard could not bring himself to use the term *X ray*, but instead employed the totally ambiguous term *wave radiation*. There is no question that Lenard believed that he deserved the fame into which he thought Roentgen had stumbled. After all, he reasoned, it was he and not Roentgen who had discovered that cathode rays could pass through an aluminum sheet covering a window he had made in a Crookes tube. Indeed, he had sent one of these tubes with an aluminum-covered window to Roentgen to begin his studies on cathode rays.

Roentgen early in 1895 did repeat Lenard's experiments, employing the Crookes tube with covered window that Lenard had sent him. Roentgen corroborated Lenard's findings that some of the cathode rays produced by a current did escape from the Crookes tube by passing through the small window. As Lenard had done, Roentgen placed a small screen coated with barium platinocyanide crystals very near the window. Its appearance when the tube was discharged was taken as proof that enough cathode rays had left the window to cause a faint fluorescence of the screen.

Having thus confirmed Lenard's findings, Roentgen began to wonder whether a window in the glass wall of the tube was necessary for the escape of cathode rays from the tube. "What if at least some cathode rays are able to pass through the glass walls of the tube?" he asked himself, and then began to find out.

He reasoned that he would have to use the screen to detect escape of the otherwise invisible cathode rays. He also suspected that fewer cathode rays would escape from the glass wall than from the aluminum-covered window; hence, the possible slight fluorescence produced in his screen might not be seen because of the bright luminescence in the interior of the Crookes tube when the current was turned on. Meticulously and patiently, he therefore covered the Crookes tube with opaque cardboard strips to obliterate all visible light. As a further precaution, Roentgen shut the curtains on all his windows so that the laboratory was in complete darkness. He then electrically excited the tube to be sure that it emitted no visible light. It did not, and he was about to begin his experiment when from the corner of his eye he glimpsed a mass of greenish-yellow color flickering very brightly in the absolute darkness, about a yard from where he was standing.

Startled by this eerie flashing, he at first thought he might have imagined the phenomenon. But when he again electrically excited the cardboard-covered tube, the flickering, flashing spurts of greenish yellow reappeared, only to disappear when the electric current was switched off. Truly mystified, he lit a match and peered at the site where the colors had appeared. He immediately spotted another screen coated with barium platinocyanide that he had left on his bench. Excitedly he switched the current to the tube on and off, on and off. Each time he switched the current on, the screen began to fluoresce, explaining in part the strange burst of colors he had been seeing.[4]

Completely unsolved was the cause of the fluorescence. That some sort of emanation was coming from the Crookes tube upon electrical excitement was clear enough, but what was the nature of this discharge? Roentgen knew that it could not possibly be cathode rays—such rays cannot travel more than several inches in ordinary air, and the fluorescent screen when he had first seen it glitter was a yard from the tube. Moreover, when Roentgen carried the screen from the bench to a new location many yards from the tube, it still fluoresced brightly when he electrically excited his tube. He sensed that he might be producing a new kind of electromagnetic wave.

On this fateful evening—November 8, 1895—Roentgen then placed a deck of cards, followed by a two-inch-thick book, between the tube and his small screen. Regardless of these objects, when he excited the tube, the screen promptly began to fluoresce. That same evening he had to be called repeatedly to come to dinner. When finally he did appear, Bertha became upset because he said absolutely nothing to her, ate almost none of the dinner, and quickly returned to his laboratory.

"What sort of ray or wave is doing what I see this one doing? Am I making some sort of mistake, or am I possibly going mad?" These were the questions torturing his otherwise wonderfully ordered mind. One thing was certain: after this November 8 happening, Roentgen forgot all about seeing if cathode rays were capable of passing through the glass walls of a Crookes tube. Now he was avidly seeking materials through which his newly discovered wave or ray could *not* pass.

He found early on that this wave, which he now designated the X ray, could not pass through lead at all and was absorbed in great part by other metals, depending on their density. Yet the ray was not absorbed by paper or wood and very little by flesh. The fact that it could pass through wood relatively unchanged intrigued him sufficiently that he placed a wooden box containing small metal weights on top of a photographic plate and then passed his X rays through the box. The result was dramatic: the film revealed only the weights, with only a mere shadow of what had been the wooden box.

It was sometime in early December, when he held a small lead pipe before a photographic plate and exposed the pipe to X rays coming from the Crookes tube, that he became awestruck and just a bit terrified. Although the plate showed the dark shadow he expected the lead pipe to produce, it also showed something he had never expected: the bones of two of his fingers that had been holding the pipe.

This disclosure that X rays could pass through his flesh and reveal his bones struck him as an almost apocalyptic revelation. "What I'm seeing is not a scientific phenomenon, it's unearthly, it's downright mystical. What will my colleagues think of these X rays that, unlike light or ultraviolet or even Hertzian waves, can reveal the most hidden parts of a human body, the bones?" he asked himself. Then and there he decided that he must share these findings with his Bertha. But he was afraid that she might doubt what he was sure he was seeing—particularly since for the last several weeks he had barely talked to her, eaten little, even slept each night in his laboratory. After a bit he hit upon a plan that he was certain would convince her that he had not become insane but had made a truly great discovery, even if it was an uncanny, unnatural one.

So one evening in December, after the two of them had finished dinner, he smiled happily and invited her to accompany him to his laboratory on the floor below. She was so glad to see him smile and eat his dinner enthusiastically, as he had not for a number of weeks, that she quickly accepted. Never before had he invited either her or their adopted daughter to visit his laboratory.

Once downstairs, he asked her to place her left hand on an unexposed photographic plate still lying in its light-proof wooden cassette. She did so, looking up rather timidly at him. He then turned on the current of the Crookes tube placed directly over her left hand, with its fourth finger bearing her gold rings.

"What's going to happen?" she asked somewhat anxiously.

"Don't worry, I'm going to turn on the current going to this glass tube. It will flash and crackle a bit, but don't let that frighten you. Just keep your left hand flat and perfectly quiet on the cassette," Roentgen reassured his timid wife as he switched on the current and let it continue for approximately six minutes. He asked her to wait while he developed the plate. He brought back the still-wet plate and handed it to her, saying, "Here's the picture of your hand that my new X ray made."

"Oh my God, I'm looking at my bones. It makes me somehow feel that I'm looking at my own death," she cried, far more terrified than pleased at what she saw.

Roentgen was overjoyed at Bertha's shocked astonishment. His X rays were *not* a phantasmal or delusional aberration of his brain, but as real as the glass walls of his Crookes tube or the cloth of the curtains at the laboratory windows. The opaque density of the two rings revealed by the X rays (see Fig. 7) aided in bringing reality to a ray whose provenance was

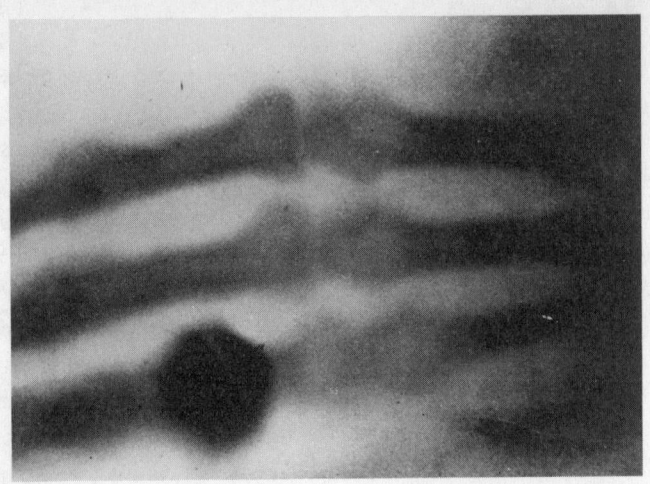

FIGURE 7. This blurred photograph is the very first X-ray print ever made. It shows the left hand of Bertha Roentgen, after a six-minute exposure to the X rays emitted by her husband's Crookes tube. Wilhelm Roentgen sent this same photograph, with a reprint of his first article, to several of his colleagues. Its publication in a Vienna newspaper was responsible for immediate worldwide awareness of the discovery of the X-ray beam.

still unknown. And unlike a light ray that can be seen, or a heat wave that can be felt, or a sound wave that can be heard, this new wave was not discerned by any of the human senses.

Immediately after he showed Bertha the X-ray picture of her hand, Roentgen decided to work in absolute secrecy. He knew, if only from this simple X-ray photograph of his wife's hand, that he had made one of history's greatest scientific discoveries. He also recognized that scores of top-notch physicists had, lying in their laboratories, Crookes tubes exactly the same as his own. If by chance one of these scientists happened to run a current through his tube in a slightly darkened room, and happened to glance at a bit of paper coated with fluorescent salts, that paper would begin to fluoresce. And if, as surely might happen, that physicist noticed the phenomenon, then Roentgen's almost miraculous discovery would be preempted.

The staid, well-balanced Roentgen became panicky. He could not breathe a word to anyone of what he was doing, and he would allow no student, colleague, or friend to enter his study except his janitorial assistant—and even *he* would not be given a hint of what Roentgen was doing. He would work as many hours of the day as he could, barely taking time to eat or sleep. For in several weeks the Physical-Medical Society of Würzburg would hold its December meeting and publish its proceedings in the society's December journal. Roentgen desperately wanted to have that issue carry a preliminary report of his X rays.

Despite his frantic rush to prepare a talk, it took him until December 28, 1895, to put together even a preliminary report. By that time the society had already convened. Roentgen nevertheless begged the secretary of the society to publish his article in December, even if he had not actually presented his report at the meeting. The secretary read the report and in all probability was ready to refuse immediate publication; after all, the journal printed only what had been presented at the most recent meeting of the society. But when his eye fell on the fourteenth of the seventeen statements constituting the manuscript, in which it was recorded that this new ray produced shadows on a photographic plate of the bones of a hand, and Roentgen showed him the X-ray photograph of Bertha's hand, the secretary knew that this report should be published immediately.

So Roentgen's preliminary report, "On a New Kind of Ray: A Preliminary Communication," appeared in the journal only a few days after he had submitted it.[5] We know of no other report of a medical discovery (not even the preliminary reports of DNA structure that appeared in the journal *Nature* twenty-two days after submission), either before or after this one, that was published within a week.

Roentgen knew that his report, published in a relatively unknown journal, would not achieve the sort of worldwide recognition he wanted. At his own expense he therefore had reprints of the article printed immediately. They were delivered to him several days before the turn of the year. On New Year's Day 1896 he sent reprints to six of the most important physicists in Europe. With them he sent copies of his X-ray photographs of the metal weights showing through the wooden box and the bones of Bertha's hand. These were telling proofs of what a truly marvelous discovery he had made. Without the photographs, physicists receiving only the reprint might have discarded his article without reading it. After all, what was so exciting about a possible new ray? Only one single phrase of the paper, as part of a long sentence describing other phenomena of the ray, intimated that the ray was able to produce a shadow of the bones of the hand.

When Franz Exner, a longtime friend of Roentgen's and now a physics professor in Vienna, received the envelope, it was not the reprint that intrigued him but Bertha's finger bones. The photograph fascinated him so much that he showed it at a party the next night—thereby both amazing and terrifying the visitors.

One of his guests was so impressed that he told his father about the photograph. The father, as it happened, was the editor of one of Vienna's most prestigious newspapers. He immediately recognized that a report of this discovery would make a fascinating, almost unbelievable story. He lost no time in getting additional details of the discovery from Exner and a complete story was splashed across the Sunday, January 5, issue of *Die Presse*. The correspondent from the *London Chronicle* immediately cabled news of the discovery to his paper, which printed its own story of Roentgen's finding on January 6. Instantly the news of the marvelous X ray appeared in newspapers throughout the world.

One of the reasons for this astounding international publicity was that the media recognized, solely from the print of Bertha's hand bones, what Roentgen himself did not fully recognize: the X ray he had discovered offered medicine an amazing diagnostic tool. Roentgen believed at first that the medical value of the X ray would be limited to possible fractures or injuries of bones.

Another reason for the immediate and vast media coverage of Roentgen's discovery was the strange uneasiness experienced by so many people that a ray had been found that was capable of penetrating their clothes and flesh to reveal their most intimate organs. It carried almost an air of indecency.[6] When X-ray photographs were first taken of the skull, they too frightened many. After all, at Halloween parties a staple decoration had always been skulls or skeletons. Moreover, for a century or more, the symbol of death had been a skull over two crossed femur bones. Indeed, in the first six months of 1896, when as a fad establishments were set up to take X-ray films of the bones of persons, many of these individuals fainted when shown their X ray–revealed bones.

As mentioned, Crookes tubes were available in scores of physics laboratories in both the United States and Great Britain. It took only weeks after Roentgen's announcement in January 1896 that a Crookes tube could instantly produce X rays for physicians in the two countries to employ X rays to visualize not only bone fractures, but bullets and any other opaque material that might have lodged in various body tissues.

It is of interest that in December 1896 an American judge declared that X-ray photographs could be admitted in court as evidence, despite the bitter objections of the lawyers defending a physician against a malpractice charge brought against him by a young law student. The student had fallen from a ladder and injured his left leg. He was advised by the physician being sued to indulge in certain exercises to heal the injury. These exercises produced such excruciating pain that the student had the leg X-rayed. The resulting photograph showed that a fracture had occurred and that the fragmented ends of the bone were not properly aligned. The misalignment probably was caused by the exercises prescribed by the physician. The law student won his case, the first of thousands of malpractice cases in which X-ray photographs have played a crucial role.

Even Kaiser Wilhelm II and his wife were fascinated by this colorless professor from the small Bavarian town of Würzburg and invited Roentgen to come to the imperial court at Potsdam. Immensely flattered, he accepted the invitation to produce and demonstrate the peculiar characteristics of the X ray. He appeared before them and their court on January 13, 1896, less than two weeks after he had mailed out his reprints. Fortunately, what he feared did not happen—the Crookes tube did not explode during the demonstration. Afterward he was invited to dine with the kaiser and members of the court. He was decorated with the Prussian Order of the Crown, II Class. Precisely why he was not decorated with the Prussian Order of the Crown, I Class, we do not know. But the decoration he did receive was good enough for Roentgen, who never forgot this stirring occasion.

On January 23 he gave the lecture to the Würzburg Physical-Medical Society that he had planned to give a month before. When he entered the Institute of Physics, he was startled and overwhelmed by the cheers that greeted him. He revealed in the lecture how surprised he had been when he discovered that the X rays were able to penetrate a deck of cards, a two-inch book, or a thick block of wood. He also confessed that it was not until he discovered that his X ray produced shadows on a photographic plate that he became certain that the wave existed and was not merely a delusion.

At the end of his talk Roentgen invited Albert von Kolliker, one of Germany's most distinguished anatomists, to come to the podium and have his hand X-rayed. The old man did so and when the audience saw the bones of his hand, it erupted in thunderous applause. Von Kolliker, commenting on the demonstration, said that during his forty-five years as a member of the society, he had never heard a presentation of greater significance in either the natural or the medical sciences.

When the meeting had concluded, a few medical scientists remained and discussed with Roentgen the possible benefits medicine might derive from X rays. The conclusion reached that evening was that because all the soft tissues of the body were of the same density, use of the X ray in medicine would be very limited. How wrong they were!

This was Roentgen's first and last formal lecture on X rays, although he was invited to speak by many organizations, including the German Reichstag. He knew that he became so flustered before any group that he actually became disoriented. Even giving physics lectures to small groups of students, he came across as lusterless, if not downright dull.

Not only did he decline to lecture to even the most distinguished audiences of the world, he also declined, with just one exception, to give interviews to newspaper and magazine journalists. He probably realized that, at an age past fifty, his days of creative research were drawing to a close. But he was determined to finish his experimental studies of the X ray, and this he managed to accomplish. His second report was published in March 1896.[7]

In this second paper he reported that X rays not only discharged "electrified bodies," they also imparted a charge to the air through which they passed. This air in turn could discharge an electrified body. The remainder of the paper described what substances could best produce X rays when impacted by cathode rays. He concluded that platinum irradiated by cathode rays was the best emitter of X rays. This second report, despite the lengthy and meticulous descriptions of the electrical properties of X rays and the metal substances most likely to emit X rays when hit by cathode rays, had nary a word about the possible medical uses of his magic waves. It was as if an archeologist, having discovered a tomb containing a mummified pharaoh with all his priceless treasures, were to present in his first report only a description of the tools employed to unearth the tomb.

Roentgen published his third and last report on X rays a year later in March 1897. Although during the year and more since he had announced his discovery physicians all over the world had taken and published X-ray photographs of fractured bones, of bullets and needles embedded in various human tissues, and of the skull and heart, in his third paper Roentgen again made no reference to the possible medical properties of his miraculous rays. He devoted the entire article to a numbing description of the physical properties of the rays and the various factors that affected those properties. Obviously disappointed, he admitted that, try as he might, he was unable to demonstrate the electromagnetic nature of the wave or its refractability—even though he somehow knew, almost certainly, that such was its nature. He had to wait seventeen years until Max von Laue discovered that the atoms in crystals were able to refract Roentgen's X ray. This wonderful demonstration by von Laue and his associates won him a Nobel Prize two years later.

Roentgen, after this third X-ray paper, published only seven more papers in the remaining twenty-six years of his life. In 1921, when he was seventy-six years of age, his last paper dealt with the effect of irradiation on the conduction of electricity in various crystals. During World War I he published nothing at all.

Although he steadfastly refused all speaking engagements, he did accept hundreds of prizes, medals, certificates, plaques, sculptures, honorary degrees, and honorary memberships in scores of scientific and medical societies throughout the world. These honors descended upon him almost immediately after his 1895 announcement. Indeed, four months after the appearance of his first X-ray article he was awarded the Royal Order of Merit of the Bavarian Crown. Roentgen accepted the decoration but refused the right to add "von" to his name. Rarely has a German scientist declined this label of nobility.

Roentgen in 1901 became the very first scientist to receive a Nobel Prize in physics. Unlike those who later came to Stockholm to receive this holy grail, Roentgen after receiving the prize from the Swedish king thanked him but gave no speech. He also did what no other Nobel laureate has done: he willed the prize money to the University of Würzburg.

After receiving the Nobel Prize, what little chance Roentgen had of doing major creative research was doomed when he was forced to leave Würzburg by Bavarian royal command to serve as director of the Institute of Physics at the University of Munich. Protest as he might, deep down (like most scientists over fifty-five who receive a Nobel Prize) it is likely that Roentgen felt relieved that he no longer would be expected to achieve wondrous research results. Working in science is never an easy task, and by no means always a pleasant one. How can any career be uniformly pleasant when disappointing laboratory results are the rule, not the exception? A real scientific breakthrough, as Sir Karl Popper pointed out, is not one that appears well confirmed, but rather one that amply provides the means by which it later can be proved erroneous.

With his new position at the University of Munich and his Nobel Prize, Roentgen became increasingly an administrator and less a researcher. He did putter sometimes in the laboratory, and of course he continued to give lectures in physics—which his students still found dull and boring.

Unlike his Prussian contemporary Robert Koch, Roentgen never attracted younger physicists as disciples. As a researcher, he was a loner. Furthermore, his social life was quite limited, perhaps owing to Bertha's chronic illnesses.

In 1903 Roentgen reluctantly accepted an invitation to deliver the keynote address at the dedication of the Munich Art Museum. The audience included leaders of the Bavarian nobility, the military, and the government. It was his first formal talk since January 1896. For some reason he panicked. He stumbled and stammered through his speech, quickly becoming so incoherent that even the journalists attending the ceremony were unable to make sense of his address. Roentgen regarded this unfortunate incident as a sheer disaster; he never again gave any sort of public lecture or address.

The essential decay of his own research activities even before the advent of World War I does not indicate that Roentgen became a vegetable, far from it. He buried himself in the directorship of the Institute of Physics and participated in many of the activities of the University of Munich, of which his institute was a part. Almost every weekend he traveled to his hunting lodge just outside Munich, where he enjoyed tracking both large and small game, and there were the annual month-long vacations in

Switzerland. Life was truly *gemütlich* for him and Bertha, nurtured as they were by their cook, maid, and housekeeper.

It thus appeared to be the best of all worlds for Roentgen—until 1914. Then the troops of his beloved kaiser invaded Belgium and set his world—and that of most other Germans—on fire. From the very first, Roentgen was queasy about Germany's prospects, despite the army's early victories in Russia and northern France. For one thing, the British blockade caused Roentgen to fear that his fatherland might not win this war.

Bertha survived the hardships of the war but died in 1919. Roentgen, then seventy-four, was still taken care of by the members of his household. The only person to whom he could open his heart and soul was the widow of the only true friend he had ever had, Leonard Boveri. But even with Mrs. Boveri, his communication was solely by letter. He did try to continue his emotional union with the dead Bertha by reading aloud, to her photograph, letters written to him years ago that he thought she might like to hear again.

On reaching age seventy-five, Roentgen retired from the university. He still occasionally went hunting but mostly took long walks. He became increasingly interested in the routine activities of his household, despite the continuing service of his three servants. In 1920 and for a long time afterward, the Germans experienced both a shortage of food and a precipitous decline in the value of the mark. Every day Roentgen had to find ways to feed and provide warmth to the members of his household. Indeed, he spent several weeks arguing with his cook and housekeeper about the purchase of a pig. They, but not Roentgen, wished to buy a small pig and raise it for butchering later. The staff won the argument. When the pig was ready to be slain, a new series of arguments began. Roentgen, who had grown fond of the pig, wanted to sell the animal but his female staff did not trust the local butcher. Rather than trade the pig for fast-depreciating marks, they wanted to kill and butcher the pig themselves, thus getting a maximal amount of scarce lard and pork. Again they won out.

Roentgen continued to receive diplomas and medals after he retired (all told, he was the recipient of well over fifty honorary doctorates and dozens of medals, many of them gold). Yet his chief joy, along with his walks, was rereading old letters to recreate past events that had thrilled him. A letter from Helmuth J. L. von Moltke reminded him of that long-ago evening of January 9, 1896, when von Moltke sat to his right and Kaiser Wilhelm II to his left at the dinner given in Roentgen's honor. That letter he read more than once to the photograph of his dead Bertha.

During the last months of 1922, Roentgen fell sick from an illness that he, but not his doctors, knew would be fatal. He died on February 10, 1923. His ashes were deposited in the family grave at Giessen, where he and Bertha had spent their happiest years.

No more honest or straightforward scientist than Wilhelm Conrad Roentgen ever lived. He literally had no discernible vices. He was a brilliant man, but his brilliance was tightly focused in that he lacked the conceptual grandeur of an Isaac Newton or an Albert Einstein. Nevertheless, when serendipity presented him with the flashing bit of fluorescing screen, Roentgen was not found wanting.

Prior to the X ray, a physician was able to employ only four of the five senses (hearing, smelling, touching, and tasting) in detecting an illness and its causes. Roentgen's discovery allowed the doctor to employ the fifth sense (seeing)—not only for detecting, but often enough for curing a disease. It is difficult even today to think of a greater gift to the physician and of course to the patient than discovery of the X ray.

It was not long after Roentgen's discovery of X rays that barium salts were found to be radio opaque. Upon being dissolved in water they were administered by mouth to visualize the esophagus, stomach, and small intestine. The same preparation introduced via the rectum allowed the large intestine to be visualized. A similar retrograde injection of an iodine solution into the ureter allowed inspection of the bladder and kidneys.[8]

Relatively harmless chemicals later were found or prepared that could be injected intravenously and, more recently, intra-arterially. Thus, for the last four decades the chambers of the heart and the interior of all the major veins and arteries of the body have been capable of inspection. But far more was still to come.

In 1972 an English computer engineer, Godfrey Hounsfield, and his colleague, a neuroradiologist, revealed for the first time the inner parts of the brain that previously had been impossible to see. The system that they employed to obtain these images, they called computerized transverse axial tomography.[9]

Hounsfield devised a system of discharging focused X rays from multiple angles and penetrating thin body slices; that is, he produced multiple tomograms. These thin-body-slice X-ray beams were converted by receptors into digitalized data, which in turn were converted by an algorithm (a special set of mathematical instructions) to construct X-ray images through use of a high-speed digital computer.

The images, first revealed at meetings of radiologists, created a tremendous stir. For the first time, intricate soft tissues and liquid chambers of the brain were visualized. The radiologists instantly recognized that with this new CT (computerized tomography) scanner not only could the various tissues of the brain be identified but so could other soft tissues of the body and their lesions.

Hounsfield almost abandoned the project in 1967, when he and his colleague, A. J. Ambrose, attempted to scan cows' heads obtained from a local butcher. The results were disappointing in that none of the intricate structures of the brain, including the ventricles, were visualized. Before they decided to give up the entire scanning project, Ambrose suggested that perhaps they had not been able to visualize the finer details of the brain because the cows whose heads they had attempted to scan had been killed by smashing their skulls. The hemorrhages ensuing in various parts of the brain might be obscuring the internal structures. Such hemorrhages possibly also filled the ventricles of the brain with blood, thus making them impossible to visualize.

Ambrose succeeded in convincing Hounsfield to go to a kosher meat market to obtain heads of cows that had been killed by cutting the great vessels of their necks rather than by battering their skulls with a heavy instrument. Sure enough, when they utilized the heads of cows bled to death by the Jewish ritual slaughterers, they obtained beautifully distinct images of all parts of the brain—including a clear picture of the ventricles.[10]

Following this critical experiment, Hounsfield and his colleagues met with the top officials of the company they worked for (E.M.I., Ltd.) and they unanimously agreed that the company should proceed to manufacture the computerized tomographic scanner.

A human head was first scanned in 1972 at a small hospital located near the E.M.I. headquarters. The scan was a total success. Within five years more than a thousand computerized tomographic scanners were in use throughout the world. Since this stunning success, Hounsfield has received many honors, including admission to the Royal Society, knighthood, and the Nobel Prize in Physiology or Medicine in 1979. Despite these well-merited honors, he still finds it difficult to overcome his trepidation when delivering public lectures. He has found some relief by first giving his speeches to monkeys or apes at zoos in the various cities where he is invited to lecture. Why this prespeech warmup helps to allay his nervousness remains a mystery to the friend who related this anecdote to us.

Allan Cormack shared the Nobel Prize with Hounsfield, because in 1963 he published an article describing the instrument he had invented, which (employing tomograms, an algorithm, and a computer) obtained remarkable X-ray images. He, however, scanned only "phantom" models, not humans. Hounsfield supposedly was completely unaware of Cormack's studies, which were published in a relatively obscure physics journal.[11]

Great as the diagnostic advantages of computerized tomography have been, the use of this complex scanner has increased enormously the cost of medical care in the United States. The machine costs well over a million dollars, and the speed of obsolescence of a given model is frightening. Unfortunately, patients are examined much too often because of the fear of most contemporary physicians: that if they are sued for malpractice (and currently one of every five American physicians can expect to be sued), the patient's lawyer inevitably will inquire whether a "CAT scan" was taken during the patient's illness or injury. Lawyers delight in harrying physicians with this kind of question, not because it is necessarily relevant, but because they believe their own medical expertise will be enhanced for the jury—or if the physician answers that no scan was performed, it may suggest to the jury that the physician is not keeping up with diagnostic advances in medicine, hence is an ignoramus. If Roentgen had lived to witness the diagnostic acumen of a computerized tomagraphic scanner, he probably would have remembered that this incredibly complex machine had its origin in 1894 when a piece of coated paper lying in his laboratory flickered when he sent a current through his Crookes tube.

7

Ross Harrison and
Tissue Culture

If you ask any tissue-culture expert today for an opinion on the work of Ross Granville Harrison, you are likely to be met by a stare and a vacant look. "Who?" Even the presidents of Johns Hopkins and Yale universities, where Harrison worked, needed some moments of reflection before they could recall what institutional memories might still exist of the man and his work.

Harrison and his discoveries are still prominently displayed in the main lobby of Johns Hopkins Hospital, however, and one of the current responsibilities of Yale's president is to appoint a new occupant of the Ross Granville Harrison professorship, a chair established in 1947 by the President and the Fellows of Yale University in Harrison's honor. It has been held by some of Yale's most distinguished biologists.

The man almost everyone seems to have forgotten made what we consider to be one of the ten most important discoveries in Western medicine.

It was tissue culture: the ability to grow living cells in the laboratory, outside the plants or animals from which they came. Harrison's discovery has made possible the study of living organisms at the cellular and even the molecular level, and the development of modern vaccines, including those for poliomyelitis, measles, mumps, and rabies. It has abetted the search for the causes of cancer (and AIDS) by providing detailed and complex biochemical information. Indeed, because of tissue culture more has been learned about the basic mechanisms of disease in the past fifty years than in the previous five thousand. And it all began with Ross Granville Harrison.[1]

Harrison was the second of five children, born in Germantown, Pennsylvania, on January 13, 1870. His mother died early, of cancer. His father was an engineer who spent a great deal of time in Russia, and Harrison was essentially raised by an aunt. He attended a school that emphasized nature study and offered field trips in the surrounding countryside, all of which stimulated Harrison's early interest in the natural sciences. On one such field trip he heroically rescued a drowning man.

His last years of schooling would take place in Baltimore. At the age of sixteen, Harrison entered Johns Hopkins University, where he was an outstanding student. He took up biology, mathematics, chemistry, Latin, and Greek, spending endless hours in the library reading the Latin and Greek classics with which he was fascinated. He earned his college degree in just three years.

Seeing the proficiency of his second child, Harrison's father encouraged him to think about graduate school, in which he enrolled at Hopkins in 1889, planning to study biology and mathematics. But in the summer of 1890 he assisted in a project involving the embryology of the oyster. It stimulated his interest so strongly that embryology became his lifelong interest.

Harrison, thus intrigued, worked for W. K. Brookes, also at Hopkins. Brookes at the time believed that the main value of the study of function in an embryo was to confirm why a particular organ or organ system developed the way it did. Harrison agreed, although he would eventually come to change his mind.

Harrison learned something more valuable from Brookes. At one point, while studying the embryology of tiny marine animals, Brookes was informed by a visitor to his laboratory that he had better hurry, since someone in France was doing the same work and would soon publish. Brookes thought for a moment, then remarked that he could never see a reason to rush research. If the French researcher did a better job, good for him; Brookes would not need to publish his own work. If, on the other hand, something was left out (which it often was), he would publish only that part of his research which complemented the French work, and that would be all that was necessary. Harrison took this philosophy with him for the rest of his life.

He went to Bonn, where he studied medicine from 1892 through 1899 — except for the year 1894, when he returned to Hopkins, wrote his dissertation, and received his Ph.D. In Bonn he met his future wife, Ida Lange, in 1893. She had just graduated from a Swiss finishing school and was fluent in English, German, Italian, and French. Harrison was fluent in English, German, and Latin, so the couple was able to converse easily in at least two languages.

When Harrison told his father he wanted to marry Ida, his father examined her family tree and approved. Ida's father, a naval person, said that it would be all right if they became engaged but they should not marry for three years. Harrison and Ida duly waited, and on January 9, 1896, they were married in Altona, Germany. Three years later Harrison received his medical degree from Bonn.

Recognizing his brilliance, Johns Hopkins appointed Harrison to its medical faculty well before he had completed his medical degree. He rose very rapidly through the academic ranks, from instructor in 1895 to associate professor the year he received his medical degree. While he was a medical student in Bonn, he was also teaching courses at Hopkins — not an easy feat in the days before the airplane. He managed to travel back and forth by ship in between the courses he was taking at Bonn and those he was teaching at Hopkins!

Harrison was fortunate in that while he was at Hopkins, Franklin P. Mall, probably the most distinguished embryologist in the world, chaired the department of anatomy. Although the relationship between the two men must have been cordial, when Mall together with the German Franz Keibel coedited their world-famous two-volume manual of human embryology, Mall amazingly never asked Harrison to contribute. This may have been because Harrison specialized in experimental embryology and did most of his studies on animals, not humans.

Harrison did not rely on his brilliance alone. He worked hard, indeed very hard, often leaving home before dawn and not returning until many hours after dark. During his first ten years on the faculty at Hopkins he published twenty outstanding articles dealing with embryology. He also founded and eventually edited 105 volumes of the *Journal of Experimental Zoology.*

From the beginning to the end of his career, Harrison was a dependable, stolid workhorse, not a lovable, charming pony. His demeanor was rather colorless and gelid. His colleagues, first at Hopkins and later at Yale, admired and respected him; yet there is little evidence that any of them (or even his children) found him warm, jovial, or inspiring. Something icy encased this great scientist.

When we talked with Elizabeth Harrison, his physician-daughter, then ninety-five years old, it was not her father whom she warmly and enthusiastically recalled, but her mother, the German-born wife of Ross Harrison. It was Ida, this graduate of a Swiss finishing school, who not only helped Harrison in many of the tedious tasks associated with his laboratory researches but bore the total responsibility of raising five children. Harrison was not the sort of father who would help his sons build structures made of Tinker Toys or construct toy houses for his daughters' dolls. As his son later bitterly recalled, his father was too busy in his career to spend time with any of the children. For Harrison, science was a domineering mistress.

It probably was in the late summer or early fall of 1906 that Harrison, still only an associate professor at thirty-six years of age, began the study that made him immortal. At this time embryologists, most of whom were taxonomic rather than experimental in their approach to the development of the embryo, were completely mystified by the processes responsible for the development of a nerve fiber. They knew that in the final development of the nervous system all nerve fibers eventually ended in or stretched out from nerve cells, but what was the origin of the long nerve fibers they saw extending in all the organs and tissues of the embryo? Perhaps the majority thought that the local tissues and organs somehow gave rise to the nerve fibers traversing their parts.

Harrison knew that microscopic observation of stained tissue-bearing nerves would never reveal what had originally formed those nerves. If only he could obtain tissue that contained nothing but nerve cells, and observe these cells as living entities for a long enough period, perhaps he would find that a nerve cell itself gave rise to a nerve fiber.

So thinking, he dissected out the medullary tube of a ⅟₇-inch-long frog embryo and immersed it under a coverslip into fresh frog lymph, which quickly clotted. Sealing the coverslip with paraffin to prevent evaporation, he continued to observe this novel preparation under the high-power objective of his microscope. As he wrote in his brief 1907 article, "When reasonable aseptic precautions are taken, tissues live under these conditions for a week and in some cases, specimens have been kept alive for nearly four weeks."[2] It was this sentence that began the science and art of tissue culture.

Harrison probably was as excited as it was possible for him to be, as he watched nerve fibers actually emerge from the nerve cells in the medullary tube and grow at a speed of 25 microns in a twenty-five-minute period of observation. He had found the answer to the provenance of the nerve fiber: it flowed from the nerve cell itself! He carefully observed the growing end of the lengthening fiber and noted that its continued growth was due to an amoeboid action of the nerve-fiber ending.

He was so obsessed with this discovery that he did not realize that although the solution to how a nerve is formed was important for embryologists, the method by which he was able to make his nerve discovery would be of infinitely more importance to mankind. Decades would pass and many other workers would enter the field of tissue culture before Harrison finally realized that this revelation of how to grow living tissue outside the body was of awesome significance.

Harrison reported his new method and his development of a nerve fiber at a small meeting of the Society of Experimental Biology and Medicine in May 1907. Unlike several of the other discoveries described in this book, Harrison's was not reported in any newspaper, only in the *Anatomical Record*.

It is highly unlikely that this May report had anything to do with Yale's offering him the chairmanship of the department of zoology and the Bronson Professorship of Comparative Anatomy, which he promptly accepted. He arrived at Yale in the fall of 1907 and remained there for the rest of his long career. Yale's president Arthur Twining Hadley wooed Harrison from Johns Hopkins with three incentives. First, he offered him a full professorship (which he did not have at Hopkins). Second, Hadley pledged that a separate department of zoology would be created. Finally, he promised that a new building would be constructed to house the classrooms and laboratories for all the biological sciences. Hadley made good on these three promises, although it required five years for the Osborn Building to be ready for occupancy by the biologists, zoologists, and embryologists who constituted the total complement of Yale's biologists.

Harrison's first few years at Yale were occupied mostly with supervision of the construction of the Osborn Building, with recruiting a new staff of scientists, and with teaching both undergraduates and graduate students.

Harrison performed the first of these tasks admirably enough. When the Osborn Building finally was completed in 1913, it was the ultimate in facilities for the teaching of students and the research activities of professional staff. The recruiting of new scientist-teachers was successful, in that the men Harrison attracted to his staff were well above the run-of-the-mill scientists of the time. But none of the scientists he recruited, and for that matter none of the graduate students he taught, ever received a Nobel Prize, much less made a discovery remotely comparable to his own 1907 discovery of tissue culture. Harrison did very poorly at the third task associated with his job, that of teaching graduate and undergraduate students. Faced with lecturing to rich, often spoiled Yale undergraduates, he actually panicked, according to the official biographer, J. S. Nicholas, who served under him for many years. His coldness, possibly his shyness, and certainly his essential colorlessness as a speaker made it almost unbearable for students to listen to his lectures. He shared the same speaking defect that we have seen afflicted Roentgen and Hounsfield.

The absorbing processes of experimental embryology prevented Harrison from exploiting the primitive and undeveloped field of tissue culture. While he continued to employ tissue-culture techniques in his embryological studies and taught visiting scientists the methods he had developed, it was the transplantation of embryonic limbs, organs, and tissue that bedazzled him for the rest of his career at Yale. Although he published several studies in which tissue culture was the methodology used, the focus of these papers was their embryological results. To be truthful, Harrison was more excited about finding that he could transplant the left embryonic limb bud to the right side of an embryo and have it develop into a typical right limb than he ever became about discovering that living tissues could exist outside the body. To Harrison, embryological observations were of tremendous importance; tissue culture was merely a tool.

In April 1917 the United States declared war on Germany. This led to an especially difficult period for Germanophile Ross G. Harrison. He had gone to a German medical school, had married a German-born woman, and had published many of his early papers in German medical journals. He was distressed that an anti-German hysteria had enveloped the American people, making them eliminate the teaching of German, changing the names of streets, parks, and even towns if these were of Germanic origin, and regarding all Germans as incipient monsters. Harrison was fearful that the Germans might have become as hysterical as the Americans and he became concerned about the safety of his daughter, Elizabeth, who was at the Bonn Medical School when the war broke out. (She was treated very well throughout the war.) Moreover, he himself was a committed pacifist. It happened that two German scientists were working in his laboratory; when both were arrested and detained, he did everything he could to protect them. These actions led to his being viewed with suspicion by many of his colleagues.

Nor was this all. In 1917 the Nobel Prize committee recommended Harrison for the prize, not for his discovery of tissue culture but for his research on the development of nervous fibers. However, because of the war, the Nobel Institute decided not to award a prize in physiology or medicine that year. Strangely enough, it did award prizes for literature, for physics, and—of all subjects—for peace (to the International Red Cross). Apparently the staff of the Nobel Institute was not impressed by the committee's choice of Harrison. He was disappointed at the outcome—not because of the prestige associated with the prize, but because of the sizable sum that accompanied the bestowal of the medal by the king of Sweden. He had hoped to be able with the prize money to send his five children to college.

After World War I ended, Harrison continued his transplantation experiments on amphibian embryos, publishing several articles a year on his transplants of limbs and other tissues in embryos. In 1925 he published his only paper on tissue culture itself.[3] It was a lackluster account containing not a hint of the future importance of his discovery.

In 1933 he was again considered for a Nobel Prize. The committee narrowed its decision to two candidates, Harrison and Thomas Hunt Morgan. A truly distinguished geneticist, Morgan opened wide the slowly expanding field of genetics, using the fruit fly as his laboratory subject. The committee in the end chose Morgan instead of Harrison, concluding that tissue culture was a technique of "rather limited value."[4] The members also decided that too many years had elapsed since Harrison's 1907 discovery—truly a senseless reason to withhold a Nobel Prize. (Happily, in 1966 the committee awarded the Nobel Prize in Physiology or Medicine to Peyton Rous, despite the fact that he had discovered fifty-six years earlier that a tumor could be caused by a virus.)

After retiring from Yale in 1938, Harrison chaired the National Research Council and played a key role not only in the history of that organization, but in the development of modern medical science. For with America's entrance into World War II the National Research Council became the workhorse of science for the federal government. This previously rather ineffectual organ of liaison between the National Academy of Science and various federal bureaus was transformed under Harrison's leadership into a diversified agency that chose scientists from all disciplines to perform the myriad tasks vital to a nation at war. For example, it was Harrison who made it possible for the British discoverers of penicillin to team up with American chemists, who found ways to produce penicillin a hundred times more rapidly than Florey and his colleagues had been able to do.

Shortly after the end of World War II, Harrison returned to New Haven. He was chosen in 1946 to give the Silliman Lectures, Yale's most prestigious scientific series. Most of his time from 1946 to 1949 was spent preparing these lectures, although he continued to publish articles on his embryological studies. Unfortunately, despite his age of eighty-five, Harrison insisted on climbing a stepladder one morning in the spring of 1955; he fell off and suffered head injuries which severely limited his activities. He died in 1959.

Had Harrison been able to read the biographical memoir of him written by Nicholas, his successor at Yale, for the National Academy of Science, surely he would have thought it a fair and succinct account of his life and career. He probably would not have observed that his memoirs portrayed a life devoted solely to work. Yet it is fitting that Nicholas ended his memoirs of Ross G. Harrison with a quotation from Psalm I "Whatsoever he doeth shall prosper."

Before Harrison's 1907 discovery of tissue culture could be recognized as one of medicine's most dazzling advances, scores of additional studies and discoveries would have to be made by hundreds of other investigators. It is appropriate that we now describe some of the more important of these developments, including some of the errors made along the way.

Alexis Carrel was born in Lyons, France, on June 28, 1873. He matriculated at the medical school at Lyons and did so well that he headed the school's department of surgery only a few years after his graduation. It was while at the medical school that in 1902 he made his most valuable contribution to medicine: successful suturing of the cut ends of an artery, an operation previously infeasible. But Carrel, fully as arrogant and irascible as Pasteur, had a difficult personality. He left France for Montreal in 1904 under a cloud, after a disagreement with the French medical hierarchy. In 1905 he moved to the Hull Physiological Laboratory at the University of Chicago.

Carrel probably was as responsible as any investigator for making known to the world that Harrison had achieved a miracle in 1907 when he found that he could grow a nerve cell outside the animal body. After hearing one of Harrison's talks, Carrel sent his assistant, Dr. Montrose Burrows, to Yale to learn more about tissue-culture techniques. While Burrows was studying with Harrison, he made marked contributions to the field, particularly his discovery that chicken plasma was a much better medium for growing tissue than clotted frog lymph.

Burrows worked with Carrel for only two years, during which they cultured tissues from embryos, adult animals, human beings, and malignant tumors. Burrows then moved to Cornell University, where he was a member of the faculty until 1915. He subsequently went into private practice in Pasadena, California, where he became interested in cancer. Though he had no prior experience, he began to undertake complex cancer surgery.

In 1942 Burrows wrote a damning letter to a friend, in which he said that Franklin Mall had told him that the whole idea of growing tissues in vitro was Mall's, that Mall himself had designed all the experiments, and that Harrison had been little more than a laboratory technician carrying out Mall's orders.[5] We know of no evidence that confirms Burrows' letter.

Carrel published his first article on tissue culture in 1911[6] and made sure that it received worldwide attention in all branches of the media. So widely did he disseminate his tissue-culture results that in 1912, one year later when he was awarded the Nobel Prize, most American scientists believed that he was given the prize for his work in that area. Many of them, belatedly discovering that it was Harrison who had founded the art and science of tissue culture, bitterly accused Carrel of having betrayed his mentor by accepting the prize that rightfully should have gone to Harrison. Harrison himself was not among those vociferously protesting; he knew that the committee had not awarded its dazzling prize to Carrel for his tissue-culture studies, but rather for his splendid discovery of how to join the cut ends of an artery and thereby avoid the complications of clot formation, constriction of the lumen of the artery, and leakage. Indeed, Harrison stoutly defended Carrel's eligibility for the prize.

Carrel did not steal the Nobel Prize from Harrison. Nevertheless, massive fraud took place in his tissue-culture laboratory, for which he must bear some of the responsibility.

Carrel first cultured chicken-heart tissue in clotted chicken plasma in 1912 and managed to get his culture to live continuously for 120 days. This was the same year he won the Nobel Prize, and his celebrity was great. Moreover, Carrel loved publicity. The *New York Times* noted, accurately, that he had managed to get a tissue culture to live for 120 days and quoted from his published work. Other newspapers were not so scrupulous. The headlines of the *Rural Weekly* of Saint Paul, Minnesota, screamed on October 24, HE KEEPS HEARTS ALIVE IN TEST TUBE AND WINS $39,000 NOBEL PRIZE.

Carrel had no sooner begun his work with tissue culture than he delegated all future studies to one Albert Eberling, who supervised a group of technicians in Carrel's laboratory and carried on the actual work. Carrel was busy lecturing and writing.

Eberling, however, changed Carrel's original technique. He took a piece of chicken heart the size of a match head (called an explant) and placed it on the floor of a glass culture vessel, together with a drop of chick blood plasma and a drop of watery extract of chicken embryonic tissue. He discovered that the extract caused the cells to grow very rapidly. The mixture clotted, but contained all the nutrients for the cells to grow, which they did. In a few days the growing cells reached the edge of the clot, having used all the nutrients available. Eberling then cut the small clot in half and put each resulting piece in a new vessel, once again adding the chicken blood plasma and the embryonic fluid. Eberling eventually claimed that he continued this division from one original explant for some thirty-four years and only threw away the last remaining cells in 1946, two years after Carrel himself had died.

Thus was born the legend of the immortal chicken heart, one of the most popular news stories of the time. The *New York World Telegram* called Carrel every New Year's Day to find out how the cell strain was doing, and published an annual editorial celebrating its birthday. In 1940 the newspaper could not reach Carrel, as he was in France, so it published a premature obituary on the chick-heart culture. Cartoonists, science fiction writers, and Sunday supplement contributors all showed a great deal of imagination in dealing with this so-called immortal chicken heart. *Collier's*, on October 24, 1936, stated that occasional trimming was necessary to keep the cell culture from growing out of the laboratory.

But this claim was far too modest. Eberling himself noted that if he had saved all the divided cell cultures, the resulting mass would have been bigger than the sun. Halving each culture each week would after twenty weeks yield one million cultures, and the number would double every week thereafter. We can see why Eberling, and others as well, kept only a few cultures at a time!

Carrel rapidly became much more famous than he had been when he won the Nobel Prize. Even today more physicians know his name, and his connection with tissue culture, than have ever heard of Ross Harrison. In 1935 he gave a series of lectures to the public, which proved so popular that police were needed to control the crowd.

Yet one of Carrel's technicians (who shall be nameless) thought something was amiss. When she looked at a clot, she noticed that the so-called immortal cells were clustered in the center. But a fraction of an inch away, she frequently saw another tiny island of living cells. She went to the chief technician and asked what process could account for the additional living cells. The chief technician told her it was not important.[7]

In 1929 the stock market crashed, the Great Depression began, and the technician realized she was lucky to have a job. But she was not happy. She had discovered that the laboratory was inadvertently introducing new live cells into the clot because of the crude way the embryonic extracts were prepared from the fresh embryos every morning. Using a balanced salt solution, she extracted the fluid from a chicken embryo with a syringe, placed it in a test tube, and spun it in a very crude centrifuge—so crude that it amounted to little more than swinging a bucket around her head once or twice. The idea was to separate out any remaining cells, so that only the embryonic fluid would feed the immortal culture. But the procedure was so crude that live cells and other cellular debris must still have been floating at random on top of the fluid. The chicken cells were not immortal after all! They were being refreshed with live cells every time they were fed.

When the assistant again brought these facts to the attention of the chief technician, he told her menacingly to be quiet if she wanted to keep her job. And she was, for thirty-three years! During that time she married and moved to Puerto Rico, where her husband became dean of the university's School of Dentistry. In the fall of 1963 she attended a lecture given by Dr. Leonard Hayflick at the University of Puerto Rico School of Medicine. During the lecture Dr. Hayflick said that, while Carrel had thought normal cells were immortal, he had himself proved they had a limited life span. He recognized that many still thought Carrel was right. After his talk, the technician walked up to him and affirmed that he was right and Carrel was wrong. Hayflick said, in his own words, "Oh my God!" and took her to have a drink, at which point she told him her thirty-three-year secret: Carrel's work was fraudulent![8]

After conversations with Dr. Jan Witkowski, who wrote an article about Carrel's chicken heart[9] and with Dr. Ralph Buchabaum,[10] who visited Carrel's laboratory and examined the chicken-heart culture, we have concluded that Carrel's preparation did not consist of immortal cells but was kept alive and growing because new chicken-heart cells were regularly added to the culture. Whether Carrel himself ever became aware of these additions cannot now be known.

Even if Carrel was essentially a publicity-seeking scientist, he did rescue Harrison's discovery of tissue culture from oblivion by his chicken-heart preparation and the wide publicity it received year after year. After his retirement from the Rockefeller Institute, he returned to France. There he became too closely bound politically to the Vichy government but died in 1944 before he could be indicted for possible political crimes.

Alexis Carrel's great achievement, and it was great, was finding a way to suture the cut ends of an artery. His work in tissue culture was at best mediocre, and at worst misled a full generation of tissue culturists and of scientists and physicians. The hurtful Carrel legend prevailed until 1959, when Leonard Hayflick, then a young postdoctoral biologist, began growing normal human cells.

The belief at the time was that only embryonic and fetal tissues were relatively free of viruses. This turned out to be largely the case, so Hayflick decided to obtain his normal cells from embryonic tissues from legal abortions, flown to him from Sweden.[11] The cells arrived at random times. Hayflick would immediately cultivate and subcultivate them. He found, however, that he could do so only about fifty times before the cells began to die. The key discovery turned out to be that those cells received eight to ten months previously were dying. Those received one, three, or six months previously were still growing vigorously, but growing in the same pool of culture medium, on the same glassware, and handled by the same technicians as the older cells. The only remaining factor, the one that caused the cells to die, was age. Hayflick's conclusion was that normal human cells were not immortal. After a number of additional studies by Hayflick and others,[12] the truth emerged: normal cells cannot divide forever.

Dr. George Gey and his wife, Margaret, of Johns Hopkins University were responsible, at least indirectly, for one of the most distressing, worldwide cellular contaminants that continues to plague not only those who work in tissue culture but also those who try to produce pure antivirus vaccines.

The catastrophe began on February 9, 1951.[13] On this day the Geys obtained a bit of tumor from the cervix of a thirty-one-year-old black woman, Henrietta Lacks. The gynecologist who removed the tissue reported that the tumor, grossly observed, did not look like the usual cancer of the cer-

vix. The tissue was red, not pale, and big blood vessels ran through it. The world-famous pathologist at Hopkins, however, labeled it a typical cancer of the cervix arising from the cells covering the cervix. Even world-famous experts can make mistakes, and later review showed that Mrs. Lacks had a cancer arising from primitive glandular, not epithelial, cells. This mistake cost Henrietta Lacks her life. Instead of radical surgery, which would have been the usual procedure, she was treated with radiation therapy, to which her particular cancer was insensitive. The cancer spread and killed her within eight months.

Unlike any other explant, her cells (subsequently called HeLa cells) grew like wildfire. They proved to be so hardy that they could be mailed anywhere in the world and survive. In fact, mail packages containing HeLa cells became famous as "HeLagrams." Samples were sent to every biomedical scientist working in the United States; they loved these cells because they grew so rapidly and so well. At first, HeLa cells appeared to be perfect for experiments.

In 1961, though, a New Jersey tissue culturist found that merely pulling a stopper from a test tube, or dispensing liquid from a dropper, was sufficient to launch airborne droplets containing HeLa cells. When these cells landed on open petri dishes containing other live cultures, they grew so vigorously that in three weeks they overwhelmed the other cells.

Then in 1966 a Seattle geneticist, Stanley Gartler, discovered an enzyme that occurred only in the cells of some black people, and of course it was present in HeLa cells as well. His discovery of this same enzyme in at least eighteen supposedly pure Caucasian cell lines in the new cell bank established in Washington, D.C., indicated that the cells of those eighteen cell lines were actually HeLa cells. They had been incorrectly classified as tumors from the liver, the blood, and other regions of the body; but all, in fact, were from the cervix of Henrietta Lacks![14]

Gartler soon read a paper on this discovery to a meeting of the members of the Tissue Culture Association. Researchers who had been working on these eighteen cell lines were furious, since, if Gartler were correct, years of their work were meaningless. The news was so shocking that for a time no one would associate with Gartler. His claims were called "wild and insolent." But the Tissue Culture Association appointed two independent research teams to evaluate all the cell lines in the national bank. Of the thirty-four, twenty-four proved to be HeLa! Gartler had been correct.[15]

The HeLa contamination and the confusion and controversy did not subside after the investigations of Gartler. The contamination of supposedly pure tissue cultures by HeLa cells was again observed by W. A. Nelson-Rees, who was in Cuba but immigrated to the United States while still a young man. Eventually he enrolled in a genetics program at the University of California, Berkeley. Receiving his doctorate in 1960, Nelson-Rees moved to a laboratory then being established in Oakland, California, by the National Cancer Institute. This laboratory was to initiate and develop a collection of new tissue cultures under the auspices of the Viral Cancer Program. Nelson-Rees became director in 1970.

He became such a perfectionist that his laboratory was far more sterile than the best operating rooms in the world. Nelson-Rees and his team were absolutely fastidious in the way they handled cells. He hired an assistant, who significantly improved the laboratory's ability to identify cells by a technique involving what is now known as chromosomal banding.[16] In addition, the laboratory routinely observed gender differences by looking for x and y chromosomes.

Apart from the war on cancer, then-President Richard Nixon was proud of his developing détente with the Soviet Union, whose scientists were persuaded to send some of their cell cultures to the United States for analysis. These were forwarded to Nelson-Rees, who found that the Russian cell cultures were in fact HeLa cells, arising from contaminated cell samples originally sent to the Soviet Union from the United States. State Department bureaucrats wanted to keep the results secret, worried that they might adversely affect détente itself. But the Soviets visited the United States and Nelson-Rees, ever the perfectionist, told them the results. The Russians, far from being upset, were delighted and invited Nelson-Rees to come to the Soviet Union. Nevertheless, every journal to which Nelson-Rees submitted his results rejected the paper, fearing the diplomatic consequences.

On another occasion Nelson-Rees discovered that five cell cultures he had been sent by various researchers were, in fact, HeLa cells. He sent a paper describing his results to *Science*, the foremost scientific journal in the

United States. One reviewer said his data were correct and another said they were extremely important, but the editor rejected the paper for no apparent reason.

One of the cell culturists whose cell line Nelson-Rees had described as HeLa contaminated, subsequently confirmed that fact on his own. He wrote to twenty researchers around the world to whom he had sent the cell line, confessing the error, with a copy of the letter to Nelson-Rees himself. Nelson-Rees resubmitted his paper to *Science*, together with the letter. This time the paper was accepted and printed, though in the very last pages of the journal.[17] Such sensational results were not ignored, however. The popular press picked up the story, and for a time it generated headlines in the United States and elsewhere.

Despite Nelson-Rees's report, many investigators continued to work with the contaminated cell lines, convinced that Nelson-Rees was wrong. Yet Nelson-Rees found that even more supposedly pure cell lines were contaminated with HeLa cells. He wrote a second article for *Science*, this time identifying the contaminated cell lines by adding the researcher's name.[18] As might be imagined, Nelson-Rees then became a widely disliked investigator.

The question of contamination with HeLa cells was not just a matter of academic debate: it had serious consequences for real people. For example, the recommendation of the maximum permissible radiation level for X-ray workers and for patients undergoing X-ray examinations derived partly from the effects of radiation on normal cell cultures. If those normal cell cultures were contaminated with HeLa cells—which, as we know, are highly resistant to radiation—then the recommendations would result in patients receiving more radiation than would be necessary or safe.

In fact, all that was known in the 1970s about the effects of radiation on tissue culture or human tissue was learned from studies of cell cultures contaminated with HeLa cells. Researchers at Pennsylvania State University in 1978 submitted an article to the prestigious *International Journal of Radiation, Oncology, Biology and Physics*,[19] in which they said that the cells they had been using were probably HeLa cells. The editor chose to eliminate that reference, calling contamination with HeLa cells "folklore." That mistake will echo and reecho for years to come.

Then in October 1978 Jonas Salk admitted that HeLa cells had overtaken the cells he had used to culture the polio virus. He had tested his vaccine on terminal cancer patients in the late 1950s. All of these patients, puzzlingly, had developed pea- to almond-sized tumors at the site of the injection. Most of the tumors had started to disappear within three weeks, but the patients generally died of their own cancers before the effects of the new tumors (probably HeLa cell tumors) could be studied. Salk and his team then discovered that the cells they had used to culture the polio virus had been contaminated with HeLa cells. But Salk announced this startling fact only after twenty-eight years had passed.[20]

Worn out by the stress he had endured since discovering the widespread HeLa contamination, Nelson-Rees voluntarily retired in 1981. A year later, probably for political reasons, the federal government closed his famous laboratory. It is estimated that the HeLa contamination Nelson-Rees uncovered has already cost taxpayers millions upon millions of dollars in totally wasted research. Unfortunately, it is probable that HeLa contamination in laboratories throughout the world continues to this day.

Back in 1953 T. C. Hsu was working in Galveston, Texas. Like other cell geneticists, Hsu could see the chromosomes in dead cells in the process of dividing. Yet they were heaped like hay in a haystack, so it was difficult to see individual chromosomes. Because of the resulting confusion, geneticists had made a grave error. They thought normal human beings had twenty-four pairs of chromosomes in each cell.

One day, as Hsu looked at the cells that had been put in a solution prepared by his technicians, he almost did a handspring. That particular salt solution was causing the cells to swell and preventing the chromosomes about to divide from forming a spindle (which is normal, but which makes the individual chromosomes hard to examine). Cells immersed in the new solution were swollen and the chromosomes were widely scattered; when fixed and stained, Hsu could observe chromosomes in detail never before seen.[21]

Hsu experimented with this new salt solution a number of times, always with the same result. The solution was an enormously valuable tool for the examination of cell chromosomes. Later Hsu took a more senior position at the famous M. D. Anderson Hospital in Houston, but to his amazement he was unable to reproduce the results he had achieved in Galveston. Puzzled, he questioned his Galveston and Houston technologists and learned that the Galveston technologists had autoclaved *tap* water, not bottled water.

Galveston, then as now, was on an island and received its water from the mainland. The pipe came in from the bay, but because it was very old and had corroded over the years, it took in seawater along with fresh water. Galveston water was almost totally undrinkable and a bottled-water industry grew up. The government of Galveston at the time was so corrupt that the bottled-water interests were able to bribe city officials not to fix the leaking pipe. Thus, what Hsu had really discovered in 1953 was the cell-swelling capacity of Galveston tap water, which to this day is used by cell geneticists the world over to treat cells to make their individual chromosomes more visible.

Hsu studied cells from a mouse, a guinea pig, a rat, a dog, and an abnormal human tumor—but not, amazingly, normal human cells. A few years later J. H. Tjio and A. Levan used Hsu's technique to study normal human cells and found that the number of human chromosomes was forty-six, not forty-eight.[22]

Hsu's technique also led to the discovery of a great number of potential chromosomal problems: people could have too many chromosomes, too few chromosomes, abnormal chromosomes (genetic counseling was one result). The technique allowed cell culturists to decide if the cells they were examining were normal or abnormal, and to check whether or not the cells were growing normally over time.

In 1958 Richard Ham of the University of Colorado became interested in culture media. Everyone in the field was using a specific cell line. Ham, noting as others had that the media used to support established cell lines were not well suited to the development of normal cells, began working to find media that *could* support the growth of normal cells.[23] He studied fibroblasts and formulated several media still in use that were named after him. In 1976 Donna Peehl, an accomplished postdoctoral student who had studied at Stanford University joined Ham's laboratory for a time. Peehl realized that the normal human epithelial cells could not grow well in the existing media. She turned to keratinocytes, a variety of epithelial cells in the skin, and decided to develop from scratch a growth medium for epithelial cells. She was able to eliminate all the previous components of media except for a tiny amount of dialyzed fetal bovine serum protein. After she left Ham's laboratory, Ham himself was able to get rid of the last serum. Thus, the two of them had developed the first entirely synthetic, entirely chemically controlled environment for the growth of epithelial cells. Ham acknowledged that Peehl's work was the first major breakthrough in the growth of epithelial cells. Since most cancers develop from epithelial cells, a way to grow them was virtually a necessity.

We have already mentioned how pleased the Delft haberdasher Antony Leeuwenhoek would have been if he could have known, two centuries after he first detected bacteria, that Robert Koch determined that one of those bacteria was the cause of tuberculosis. Unlike Leeuwenhoek, Ross Harrison did have the keen satisfaction of knowing that his little 1907 paper had led to one of medicine's greatest triumphs: successful tissue-culture growth of one of mankind's most vicious viruses, that of poliomyelitis.

Long before Harrison devised tissue culture, several vaccines made of viruses had been used to prevent the onset of the diseases caused by these viruses. We have already described the cowpox vaccine, whose administration has wiped out smallpox. We have described Pasteur's employment of the attenuated rabies virus to prevent the onset of malignant rabies in man. Why, then, did medicine stand by helplessly and watch bulbar poliomyelitis kill or cripple hundreds of thousands of children and young adults? The answer is simple: medicine had not yet found a reliable way to grow the virus causing the disease. The poliomyelitis virus, like all other viruses, can exist and proliferate only in living cells.

The virologist Albert Sabin and his colleagues claimed in a preliminary report in 1936 that they were able to grow a polio virus.[24] Today there is considerable doubt that their virus was living. It was certainly incapable of the kind of viral proliferation that would furnish enough virus for production of a vaccine. In any event, Sabin performed no further studies on this embryonic tissue preparation. Instead, he publicly pronounced, in his ex cathedra way, that polio viruses would never grow in tissue culture.

This statement did not discourage John F. Enders. After receiving his doctorate from Harvard University in 1930, he stayed there for the remainder of his career. He began working on viruses and their tissue culture in 1939, and eight years later was invited to set up an infectious diseases laboratory in the Harvard-affiliated Children's Hospital in Boston. Two years later he and his two postdoctoral fellows, T. H. Weller and F. C. Robbins, sounded the death knell for poliomyelitis. They had found a way to grow the deadly virus in tissue culture.[25]

In this modest two-page article, Enders demonstrated that he and his colleagues were able to propagate the polio virus not only in neural tissue but in muscle and intestinal tissue. This finding was of tremendous importance, because later it was determined that when the virus was grown in extraneural tissue it lost its virulence for humans yet retained its vaccinating power.

These two pages from Enders and his colleagues brought real joy to Ross Harrison, now almost eighty years of age. At long last, forty years after his monumental discovery, he knew it would result in vaccines that would prevent major viral epidemics such as poliomyelitis, measles, mumps, whooping cough, and chicken pox. Salk and his associates in 1953 reported the protective power of a vaccine composed of inactivated polio virus particles that had been obtained by growing the polio virus in tissue culture, as made possible four years earlier by Enders and his colleagues.[26] Sabin's vaccine, consisting of live but inactivated virus, was licensed in 1960. As a result of these two vaccines, it is quite probable that by 2010 poliomyelitis will no longer exist on our planet.

Harrison was still alive in 1954 when Enders, along with Weller and Robbins, were given the Nobel Prize in Physiology or Medicine "for their discovery of the ability of poliomyelitis virus to grow in cultures of various types of tissue." That his two young colleagues (at the time of the discovery only postdoctoral fellows) be included was Enders' idea. A true gentleman, he insisted that they be recognized as well as himself. Harrison, twice nominated for this same prize, was totally delighted that it was awarded to Enders and his associates. No one knew better than Harrison that it was his 1907 observation of a nerve fiber living and growing in frog lymph that had led to this magnificent triumph!

8

Nikolai Anichkov and Cholesterol

Ask any zoologist or epidemiologist what animal has killed and is still killing more humans than any other animal. The answer would surely be the cobra. Despite the availability of antivenom therapy, this wretched snake still kills five thousand to ten thousand Indians alone each year. A herpetologist would incriminate not the relatively long (10–15 feet) king cobra, but the short (5 feet) Indian snake (naja naje). This reptile ranks as the most deadly because of its habit of slinking into houses at dusk in search of rats and mice, then being surprised by an unsuspecting human victim, into whom it buries its lethal fangs.

The specialists would be in error. The most murderous animal for millennia has been and still is the seemingly gentle hen. She does not kill us by fang or claw but by presenting us with the product of her ovary. The yolk of her egg contains ten times as much cholesterol as is found in a similar quantity of beef, pork, fish, or even chicken flesh. No other body organ or tissue (except the brain) is so loaded with this lethal substance.

And unlike the brain, which is ingested rather sparingly by civilized man, egg yolk infiltrates our soups, our sauces, our pastries, our breads, our pastas, our ice creams, and even our beverages (think of milk shakes and eggnogs). A modern chef who happened to lose a right arm could still create gourmet foods; if deprived of the use of egg yolks, that individual still might serve edible preparations, but with a broken heart.

In this chapter we shall relate how examination of the chicken egg led to recognition of the deadliness of cholesterol. We also shall try to clarify why this discovery, made more than eighty years ago, still is not totally accepted by all scientists.

Millions of persons, as far back as mummified Egyptians, have died of arteriosclerosis, a disorder blocking their coronary arteries, their cerebral arteries, or the arteries to their viscera. For many centuries this disorder did not receive any scientific attention. Even when the great English physician Caleb Parry in 1799 published his discovery that angina pectoris was due to obstructed coronary arteries, it drew little attention.[1]

During the nineteenth century, interest in this matter of arteriosclerosis increased, but real research was stymied because there were three different views on the cause of the disorder. The first and most dominant was that arteriosclerosis was simply a senescent process and not a disease at all. The second view, promulgated by Rudolf Virchow, the dominant leader of pathology for most of the century, was that arteriosclerosis was indeed a disease, but it sprang from some disturbed metabolism of the artery itself.[2] The third view, vigorously defended by the pathologist Karl Rokitansky, was that the arteriosclerotic process evolved from clots adhering to arteries, which gradually changed into typical arteriosclerotic plaques.[3]

These three contrasting theories so preoccupied their adherents that none of them even tried to approach the problem experimentally, by reproducing the disorder in an animal. They contented themselves with looking at arteriosclerotic arteries with their naked eye or with their microscope.

Besides the debate about the cause of arteriosclerosis, there was deeper confusion about which layer of an artery was initially involved in the pathogenesis. Some believed that the process began in the inner lining or intima of the artery, whereas others claimed that the process involved primarily the middle, muscular coat of the artery. And there were those pathologists who insisted that it was the outer coat or adventitia of the artery that was the initial site of the arteriosclerotic process.

The first genuine advance was made by F. Marchand, who introduced the term *atherosclerosis* to describe the disturbance that he was certain began in the inner lining of the artery.[4] He differentiated this lesion from any that began in other coats of the artery. More important, he pointed out that it was this atherosclerosis that was responsible for almost all obstructive processes in the arteries. The first hint that cholesterol might be involved in the pathogenesis came when A. Windaus reported in 1910 that atheromatous lesions contained six times as much free cholesterol as a normal arterial wall, and twenty times more esterified cholesterol.[5]

These last two studies, important as they were in retrospect, did not lead to discovery of the major cause of atherosclerosis. That resulted from four studies performed by a tiny cluster of young Russian physicians, all working at the same medical school, focusing their attention on the supposedly harmless chicken egg.

Before we describe their work, let us first examine the life of the man who was the driving force behind this congeries of previously unknown Russian physicians. The man was Nikolai Anichkov, an aristocratic Russian who was born in Saint Petersburg on November 3, 1885. On the paternal side his lineage was a distinguished one, in that the first Anichkov was a Tartar Mongol who in 1301 was baptized. The great-grandfather of Anichkov was ennobled in 1746, and throughout the nineteenth century most family members served as officers in the czar's army. Nikolai's father, however, was a minister of education, a senator, and later a member of the state council in Saint Petersburg. His mother, born in France of Russian parents, was involved in affairs of the Russian Orthodox church. It is probable that her progenitors were not of the Russian aristocracy. She was a decent woman who was totally devoted to the needs of her husband and his brother.

The first indication that Anichkov might be more than an ordinary person was his 1903 graduation from his gymnasium with a gold medal. Immediately afterward, he applied for and gained admission to the imperial Military Academy of Medicine in Saint Petersburg, the oldest and most distinguished medical school in Russia. He did very well and finished the undergraduate phase of his medical education in 1909. He continued his medical studies at the academy, working in the pathology department, and received his doctorate in 1912.

Fortunately for Anichkov, a clinician (A. I. Ignatowski) at his medical school tried in 1908 to do what no other investigator had ever attempted, namely, to induce atherosclerosis in an experimental animal. He chose rabbits, feeding them a mixture of eggs and milk. How excited he must have been to note, after a few weeks of feeding his rabbits this diet, that their aortas exhibited the same grayish-white plaques observed in the aortas of human beings. For the first time then he had reproduced a facsimile of the common human atherosclerotic plaque.

Ignatowski wrongly believed that the atherosclerosis he had produced was caused by the protein in both the milk and the eggs. He published these findings,[6] but for some reason did not continue his studies.

These results were not lost on Anichkov and his subordinates in the pathology department. Probably at Anichkov's suggestion, a young member of the department, N. W. Stuckey, repeated Ignatowski's experiment— except that he fed his rabbits three different supplements. The first group received a muscle fluid supplement; the second group, an egg white supplement; and the third group, only egg yolk. Stuckey found that only the aortas of the rabbits fed egg yolk exhibited atherosclerotic plaques. This finding made it clear enough that it was not the feeding of protein, as Ignatowski had believed, that caused the atherosclerosis. It was some dire substance in the yolk of a chicken's egg that was responsible for the onset of one of man's most devastating afflictions.[7]

"We need to determine what component of that yolk is responsible for its disease-producing potential," the young Anichkov must have thought— because on learning of Stuckey's findings, he immediately decided to feed egg yolks to rabbits and then analyze the atherosclerotic plaques to see if any particular chemical substance was concentrated in them.

Because Anichkov himself was occupied with finishing his study of diseased hearts (the topic of his doctoral dissertation), he delegated to another student under his tutelage the task of feeding rabbits egg yolks and then examining the aortic atherosclerotic plaques that appeared. The student, S. Chalatov, on examining his yolk-fed rabbits, observed a very interesting phenomenon. Their plaques teemed with what appeared to him to be lipid (fatlike) droplets that were doubly refractile and under polarized light showed beautiful double-cross figures. Also, the livers of these rabbits were overloaded with the same lipid droplets.[8]

Both Chalatov and his mentor, Anichkov, were well aware of the fact that cholesterol possessed these physical qualities; they were aware too that another chemical substance, phospholipid, which was also abundant in egg yolks, had the same properties. Further, it was possible that the lipid droplets arose from deterioration of the aortic wall or the liver.

It is likely that Anichkov and Chalatov, on seeing these results, were fairly certain that the cholesterol in the yolk was responsible for the atherosclerosis that promptly occurred when the yolk was fed to rabbits. So suspecting, they fed rabbits a pure cholesterol supplement and after a few weeks the rabbits were sacrificed. Their arteries were examined. What the two men found and reported in 1913 was one of the ten greatest discoveries of Western medicine: they discovered that cholesterol, far from being harmless, was actually the primary factor in initiating atherosclerosis.[9]

Following this discovery of the atherogenic capacity of ingested cholesterol, Anichkov was awarded a traveling fellowship. He went to the laboratory of Ludwig Aschoff, who at the time was considered the most accomplished of all German pathologists. Anichkov had been in Germany for fourteen months when World War I broke out; he faced imprisonment because of his Russian nationality. Directly aided by Aschoff, he was able to escape to Switzerland and from there to Saint Petersburg, where in 1914 he joined the faculty of the Military Academy of Medicine. He entered the Russian Army Medical Corps in 1916 and served as medical director of a military medical train. In 1917 he joined the Bolshevik Party and remained a loyal Communist for the rest of his life.

In 1920 he was appointed director of general pathology at the academy's medical school in Saint Petersburg, a position he held until his death in 1964 of a myocardial infarction. He participated in many different medical studies, including twenty-year investigations of infectious diseases, wound healing, and the reticuloendothelial system. In 1939 he was elected to the Russian Academy of Science, the most prestigious scientific organization in the country. There was little question that he had become recognized in Russia as its most gifted pathologist, a reputation that did not stem solely from his studies of cholesterol. He made other contributions to pathology, particularly those dealing with a system of peculiar cells found chiefly

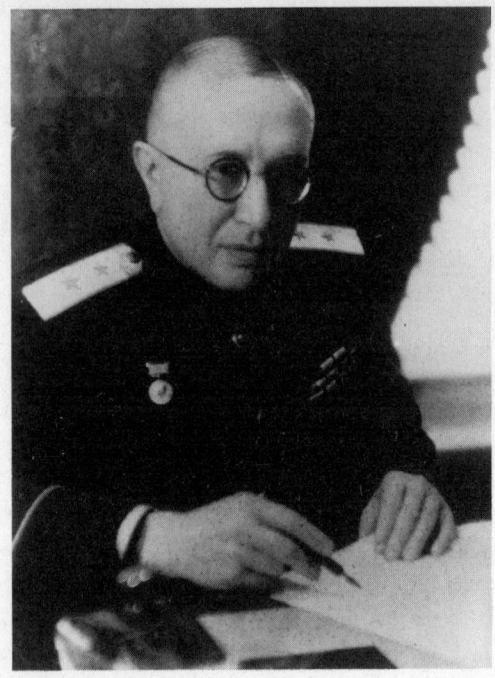

FIGURE 8. A 1945 photograph of Lieutenant General
Nikolai Anichkov of the Russian Army Medical Corps.
(Photograph courtesy of Anichkov's grandson,
Professor Nikolai Anichkov of Saint Petersburg.)

in the capillaries of the liver and spleen, cells whose exact role still has not been elucidated completely.

Throughout his medical career he remained a loyal, indeed doctrinaire, member of the Communist Party and a friend of Joseph Stalin. In 1941, he and the entire staff of the Military Academy of Medicine were transferred from Leningrad to the far safer Samarkand, where he remained for the duration of the war. In 1945 he was made a lieutenant general, the highest obtainable rank in the Army Medical Corps (see Fig. 8).

Anichkov returned in 1945 to Leningrad, where he resumed his position as director of general pathology at the academy. It should be emphasized that despite his involvement in World War I and World War II, in the political activities of the Communist Party, and the various pathological studies he had to supervise as director of the pathology department, he never lost interest in the 1912 discovery that ingested cholesterol induced atherosclerosis in the rabbit (and also in the guinea pig). He managed, in a period between the two world wars, to extend his investigation of this subject.

He somewhat altered his views in 1924, proposing what he termed a combination theory concerning the etiology of atherosclerosis. Anichkov admitted that the feeding of cholesterol was not the sole cause of human atherosclerosis. He stressed that at least 10 percent of rabbits fed large amounts of cholesterol still never exhibited atherosclerosis and never showed a rise in their blood content of cholesterol (that is, they never became hypercholesterolemic). This fact led Anichkov to declare that just feeding cholesterol was not enough to induce atherosclerosis — the rabbits must also become hypercholesterolemic.

He also admitted that in human atherosclerosis, hypertension as well as inflammatory processes directly involving the inner lining of the artery might accentuate the atherosclerotic process. Yet Anichkov insisted on the core role of ingested cholesterol in inducing atherosclerosis. Despite his numerous publications in the 1950s, he remained relatively unknown to European and American scientists. Perhaps the lack of international recognition stemmed from his disinclination to become well recognized outside Russia. One need only peruse his Slavic face, with its high forehead and cheekbones, to recognize it as the visage of a man who was neither gregarious nor benevolent. Indeed, his was the face of a full-fledged Communist of 1918 Bolshevist provenance. It might remind one of a judge's countenance as he pronounced not a death sentence, but a prison term of twenty years. In sum, it was the face of a man not cruel, but not easily given to compassion.

Nevertheless, one might ask why a discovery of such monumental importance was ignored by the majority of the medical profession until the past several decades. Even in the 1990s there remain investigators who are far from convinced of the danger of eating eggs and other foods rich in cholesterol.

There are several reasons for this tragic lag in recognition. First, Anichkov, although always able to induce atherosclerosis in rabbits and guinea pigs by adding cholesterol to their diet, totally failed to induce the same arterial process in rats, no matter how much cholesterol they were fed.

Similarly dogs' arteries remained healthy regardless of how much cholesterol they received. Anichkov explained these exceptions by noting that neither of these animals became hypercholesterolemic after ingesting cholesterol. He commented too that, unlike rabbits and guinea pigs, dogs and rats partook of an omnivorous, not a vegetarian, diet. These facts of course initially made him wonder whether his findings in rabbits would have relevance to humans, whose diet, like that of rats and dogs, was omnivorous. If he had been able to induce atherosclerosis in rats and dogs in 1912, his doubts about the role of ingested cholesterol in inducing atherosclerosis in humans would have vanished. But more than thirty years had to pass before A. Steiner and F. E. Kendall demonstrated that, under certain circumstances, they were able to induce hypercholesterolemia and a resultant atherosclerosis in dogs by feeding them dietary cholesterol in abundance.[10] To this day, rats cannot be made hypercholesterolemic or atherosclerotic no matter how much cholesterol they are fed.

A second reason for the failure of Anichkov's discovery to be recognized and acted upon by Western investigators was the fact that no mainstream scientists concerned themselves with the etiology or pathogenesis of aortic or coronary atherosclerosis. The electrocardiograph was not in general clinical use until the middle of the 1920s; even the occurrence of a heart attack was rarely diagnosed, again until the mid-1920s. So although Anichkov's recognition that the feeding of cholesterol led to atherosclerosis in the rabbit was confirmed by isolated investigators such as C. H. Bailey in 1916 and Timothy Leary in 1935,[11] the discovery was essentially ignored. It did not help matters that one of America's most distinguished clinicians, Soma Weiss, teamed up with Nobel laureate George Minot to write an article belittling the pathogenic importance of dietary cholesterol.[12] That neither author had ever been involved in relevant studies did not deter them in the least.

Other reasons too may have contributed to the nonrecognition of Anichkov's discovery for forty years. Lord Byron once wrote to Goethe congratulating him on his good fortune that his name was easy enough to be articulated by posterity. Byron could hardly have congratulated Anichkov on the simplicity of *his* name. Those who bear names that are difficult both to spell and to pronounce are relatively unlikely to be remembered by succeeding generations, regardless of their achievements. Then, too, Anichkov was totally unknown to European and American scientists, and his medical school, distinguished as it probably was to Russians, was unknown as a research center to Western investigators.

Similarly, the Russian language is not a lingua franca for the scientists of any country, and almost all the writings of Anichkov and his colleagues were published in Russian. The only reference to his cholesterol discovery in the American medical literature was a chapter written by Anichkov for the first edition of E. V. Cowdry's book *Arteriosclerosis: A Survey of the Problem*, published in 1933, and a similar chapter appearing in the second edition in 1967, three years after Anichkov's death.

This failure of Anichkov's discovery to be exploited by other scientists does not mean that there were no suspicions about cholesterol in the 1930s and 1940s. Determinations of the blood concentration of cholesterol commenced in the 1930s, and persons with an excess of this substance in their blood were advised to avoid eating cholesterol-rich foods, especially eggs. Then, in the 1950s, two separate discoveries and an editorial led to renewed interest. Today the field is crowded with thousands of investigators studying every facet of the role of cholesterol in the pathogenesis of atherosclerosis.

The first of the three "breakthroughs" was a 1950 article of John Gofman and his associates in *Science*.[13] Theirs was the first study ever published by this most prestigious of all American scientific journals to deal with cholesterol as an artery-damaging substance.

Gofman began by emphasizing that it was Anichkov who first showed that the feeding of cholesterol to rabbits promptly led to atherosclerosis in this animal. Employing his technique, the Gofman group had confirmed that Anichkov was correct; their cholesterol-fed rabbits promptly exhibited atherosclerosis. Then they were able to do something that Anichkov could not have done in 1912: they developed an ultracentrifuge capable of rotating its tubes forty thousand times per minute. No previous centrifuge had possessed such rotating capacity. Their machine obtained it by both refrigerating the rotating tubes and evacuating air from the space in which the tubes were rotated.

When the hypercholesterolemic serum samples of their cholesterol-fed rabbits were introduced into this fantastic ultracentrifuge, their cholesterol content was found to be sequestered in two distinct compartments.

The first of the two fractions, which they designated the low-density lipoprotein cholesterol, floated toward the surface of the serum samples. The second cholesterol-carrying complex, which they designated the high-density lipoprotein cholesterol, was deposited at the bottom.

The low- and high-density lipoprotein cholesterol fractions basically carried the same molecules (cholesterol, protein, phospholipid, and triglyceride), but the low-density fraction was richer in triglyceride content and lower in protein (which was responsible for its low density) than the high-density complex. The Gofman group also observed that whereas the cholesterol in the blood of normal rabbits was carried almost exclusively in high-density lipoproteins, in strong contrast, most of the cholesterol in the cholesterol-fed atherosclerotic rabbits was chiefly carried in the low-density lipoprotein complexes.

After detecting this low-density lipoprotein cholesterol molecule in rabbits made hypercholesterolemic and atherosclerotic by the feeding of cholesterol, Gofman and his coworkers examined with their marvelous ultracentrifuge the blood serum of 104 male patients who had recovered from a heart attack (due of course to underlying coronary atherosclerosis) and 94 normal male subjects. The blood serum of 101 of the 104 coronary atherosclerotic men abounded in large fractions of the same low-density lipoprotein molecules they had observed in their cholesterol-fed, atherosclerotic rabbits. On the other hand, they found almost none of this same molecule in the serum of the normal young men. Similar findings were observed in female subjects with and without coronary disease.

The Gofman group also found that while hypercholesterolemic men did exhibit a high concentration of this low-density molecule, it also could be observed in men with normal total blood cholesterol content. They argued that this finding would explain why a fairly large fraction of men who suffered an infarction had a normal or even a low *total* blood cholesterol content. They did admit that feeding of cholesterol to individuals already carrying this low-density molecule in their blood would increase its concentration still more.

Publication of the Gofman article literally awakened the medical and lay community to the perils of dietary cholesterol. The introduction of a complex technical instrument, the ultracentrifuge, for help in investigating a medical problem attracted the widespread attention of the media, if only because it was the first major contribution of physics to medicine since Roentgen introduced his X-ray machine in 1895.

Then too, the seeming identification of a specific sort of cholesterol (low-density lipoprotein cholesterol) rather than generic cholesterol as an atherogenic agent appeared to explain why so many persons suffered heart attacks even though their total blood cholesterol was lower than the accepted normal levels.

These findings, so widely publicized in the media, irritated some old-line cardiologists. While believing that cholesterol did play a significant role in bringing on coronary heart disease, these physicians nevertheless scoffed at the idea that only a certain sort of lipoprotein cholesterol was the guilty substance. The Gofman group, almost arrogant in its insistence that the quantity of low-density lipoprotein cholesterol in the blood — not the total cholesterol — determined the cardiac fate of Americans, proposed an epidemiological study in which the blood of thousands of Americans still free of heart disease would be analyzed for its total as well as its low-density lipoprotein cholesterol content. This large group would be followed for a number of years to determine whether the future heart attacks that would occur in some of these volunteers were best forecast by the blood level of their *total* cholesterol or by their low-density lipoprotein cholesterol content.

All sorts of national committees were formed to serve as referees for this widely publicized study. Dozens of the dazzling ultracentrifuges were employed to measure the low-density lipoprotein cholesterol fractions of the blood of all participants. Acrimony soon made its appearance, and the Gofman unit publicly complained about the measurements made by those who believed that the predictive value of total cholesterol content would prove to be as good or better than the low-density lipoprotein cholesterol content of the blood. So a new referee committee, headed by the eminent cardiologist Paul Dudley White of Harvard, was created.

As so often happens in epidemiological studies, the results appeared to be equivocal. Persons possessing a high total cholesterol content were about as liable as persons harboring a high blood content of low-density lipoprotein cholesterol to succumb to a future infarction. Despite the seeming parity in the prognostic capability of the two forms of cholesterol that resulted from this poorly managed study, most investigators were aware that when the total blood cholesterol was elevated, the cholesterol responsible for this elevation was mostly low-density rather than high-density lipoprotein cholesterol. This seemed to suggest that a high content of low-density lipoprotein cholesterol was potentially atherogenic.

For about a decade not much attention was paid to the manner in which cholesterol was carried in the blood. But simple chemical methods for analysis of the lipoprotein cholesterol fractions replaced the expensive ultracentrifuge, thus allowing almost all clinical laboratories to perform this analysis. With new epidemiological studies being performed in the 1960s and 1970s, the potential danger of low-density lipoprotein cholesterol was "rediscovered." Today, although most workers in the field of atherosclerosis refer to low-density lipoprotein cholesterol as the "bad" cholesterol and high-density lipoprotein cholesterol as the "good" cholesterol, very few remember or refer to the pioneering findings of John Gofman and his associates.

The second breakthrough of the 1950s that led to thousands of new cholesterol studies was the discovery in 1952 by Lawrence Kinsell and his group that ingestion of plant foods and avoidance of animal fats significantly decreased the blood level of cholesterol in most humans. This study was confirmed by E. H. Ahrens and his colleagues, who learned also that the cholesterol-lowering effect of ingesting vegetable fats was due to their relative unsaturation.[14]

Kinsell's paper led to the contemporary situation in which millions of Americans try to substitute vegetable for animal fats in their diet. This still-expanding tendency has resulted in the multibillion-dollar growth of industries offering foods rich in unsaturated fats.

Kinsell did not fare well for too long after his pioneering study. He had always believed in using only humans for his studies, and his subjects occupied about ten hospital beds as they ingested the vegetable and fruit diets. Unfortunately, there was an acute shortage of beds in the county general hospital in Alameda, California, where he worked. The administrators of the hospital, and probably the majority of its physicians, were not sufficiently impressed by Kinsell's study (despite its confirmation) to continue to allocate hospital beds to him. Simultaneously, possibly because he had carried on his experimental work in a hospital totally unknown for scientific contributions, he was not successful in obtaining grant support from any foundation.

Deeply depressed by these research disasters, Kinsell one morning phoned his secretary and told her to come immediately to his home. When she did so, she discovered the dead bodies of Kinsell and his wife. Both had taken cyanide.

It would be fitting if one of the large corporations now making millions of dollars from the sale of their various vegetable-fat products would sponsor a fellowship bearing Kinsell's name. At present there is nothing to remind us of his existence except his momentous 1952 publication.

The third event in the 1950s that awakened scientists and clinicians alike to their fifty-year neglect of the possible relationship of dietary cholesterol to coronary artery disease was not a laboratory study but an extraordinary editorial that appeared in 1958 in *Circulation*, the official publication of the American Heart Association.[15] The editorial was written by William Dock, who at the time was chairman of the pathology department at Stanford University Medical School.

The editorial was outspoken, flamboyant, and as pleonastic as Dock himself. He roundly chastised cardiac researchers for their half-century of neglect of Anichkov and his colleagues. Dock considered Anichkov's results to be of such importance that he remarked in his editorial, "Thus the early work of Anichkov bears comparison with that of Harvey on the circulation and of Lavoisier on the respiratory exchange of oxygen and carbon dioxide." Such a tribute might be somewhat overblown, but Dock in this editorial did not hesitate to employ exaggeration and scorn. For beyond the failure of researchers to take notice of the findings of Anichkov and his colleagues, they had also neglected thirty or more reports that appeared after the Russian studies. All shared one common finding: dietary cholesterol plays a key role in making arteries — whether large or small — atherosclerotic.

As a result of these landmark discoveries of the Gofman and Kinsell groups, and Dock's consummate summary editorial, hundreds of investigators (primarily American) began to take a real interest in the pathophysiology of cholesterol. In the 1960s and 1970s the pathways by which cholesterol is absorbed from the intestine, its passage from the intestine to the blood via the thoracic lymph duct, and its final absorption from the blood by the liver were discovered. In addition, the synthesis as well as the destruction of cholesterol by the liver were revealed.

It also was determined that the blood level of cholesterol is not determined solely by the dietary intake of this substance. In 1958 it was learned that emotional stress could have a profound influence on the blood level of cholesterol.[16] In 1983 M. S. Brown and J. L. Goldstein discovered that the key mechanism for the control of the blood cholesterol level probably resides in several types of lipoprotein cholesterol receptors lying chiefly in the surface membranes of cells of the liver. Here these so-called receptors control the rate of exit from the blood of the various lipoprotein cholesterol molecules. The function of these receptors, while chiefly genetically determined, can be influenced by certain of the body's hormones and by drugs.[17]

Besides these multiple studies concerning cholesterol, scores of studies are under way on the coronary arteries themselves. Anichkov himself recognized in his final paper that local changes in the inner lining of the artery could significantly influence the atherosclerotic process.[18]

Secure as all these laboratory advances have been, only inconclusive results have been attained in attempts to determine whether the ingestion of cholesterol by a large group, or even a total population, correlates with the coronary mortality suffered by these same groups or populations. While such studies have given employment to hundreds of medical and paramedical personnel, their findings can at best be described as ambiguous. So confusing and contradictory have these vast multimillion-dollar epidemiological surveys been that so-called meta-analyses were initiated by new groups of epidemiologists. The disparate results of dozens of earlier population and group studies were summarized, to determine whether there were any conclusions on which at least the majority of these prior epidemiological studies agreed. But most of these meta-analyses have proved worthless also.

The fundamental error in these group and population surveys has been their failure to take into account variables that cannot be measured and fed into computers. For example, a considerable number of factors besides the amount of dietary cholesterol ingested may increase the coronary death rate in various groups of people. For example, psychological factors that have recently been recognized as coronary risk factors were completely ignored by past epidemiological studies. This costly mistake was made not solely because such factors are not easily measured in units acceptable to computers, but also because of the lack of awareness of epidemiologists themselves of the clinical and sociological characteristics of coronary patients. After all, if one works long enough with computers, one starts to think like a computer.

Today most cardiologists are convinced that Anichkov was correct in insisting that dietary cholesterol does induce atherosclerosis. But they also believe, as did Anichkov later on, that other factors play a part in finally closing a coronary or cerebral artery. Emotional stress, hypertension, cigarette smoking, inborn or genetically determined errors in lipoprotein cholesterol cell receptors, and diseases such as diabetes all may play a part in producing atherosclerosis. Anichkov was essentially correct, though, in insisting that the ingestion of cholesterol is the prime factor in inducing the most deadly of man's present disorders. The tragedy has been that unlike Roentgen's discovery of X-rays, which was recognized in weeks as a tremendous discovery, Anichkov's discovery was unnoticed for many decades. Even today, while it is true that man does not live by bread alone, he and his partner are more than a little reluctant to avoid ingesting eggs and the many other foods containing cholesterol.

9

Alexander Fleming and Antibiotics

In 1875 John Tyndall, England's most distinguished physicist, was busily engaged in trying to find out whether bacteria were evenly dispersed in the atmosphere or aggregated in "clouds." If they were evenly distributed, Tyndall reasoned that if he set up a number of open test tubes containing broth, all the tubes should become turbid from the growth of bacteria falling into them from the air. But if bacteria were amassed in clouds, then only some of the culture tubes would be contaminated.

With this plan in mind, he set up one hundred open test tubes containing broth, placed a moderate distance from each other. When he examined the tubes the next day, the broth in a number of them remained clear, indicating that no bacteria in the air had fallen into these tubes. The implication was that bacteria were not evenly dispersed in the atmosphere.

Twenty-four hours after he had exposed the tubes, Tyndall observed something infinitely more important. Lying on the surface of the broth in some of the tubes was a *Penicillium* that was "exquisitely beautiful." A battle was also under way between the bacteria and the mold, and "in every case where the mold was thick and coherent, the bacteria died or became dormant and fell to the bottom as a sediment."[1]

One might ask why Tyndall, having observed that this exquisitely beautiful mold (which we now know was *Penicillium notatum*) was capable of destroying bacteria, contented himself with remarking on its physical beauty and its bacteriocidal capacities without exploring the second phenomenon further.

The reason is clear. He discovered the antibacterial property of the *Penicillium* seven years before Robert Koch in 1882 proved that bacteria could cause disease. If Tyndall had known that most infectious diseases were caused by bacteria, it is extremely unlikely that he would have continued to interest himself in the possible cloudlike array of bacteria in the atmosphere. Rather, he would have immediately revealed his observations to his medical friends. Not knowing that bacteria caused infections, he was content to limit his observations to a few brief sentences that were buried in a seventy-four-page article describing the disposition of bacterial and other particles in the atmosphere.

Other than a report in 1896 by a young French medical student, stating that animals inoculated with both *Penicillium glaucum* and virulent bacteria fared far better than animals receiving virulent organisms alone,[2] and the publication of a short note in 1925 by D. A. Gratia of the University of Liège describing his observation that a substance produced by a *Penicillium* mold could dissolve anthrax bacilli, essentially fifty-four years would elapse, and millions of preventable deaths would occur, before the antibacterial power of this same species of *Penicillium* would be rediscovered.

During this long delay in the rediscovery of penicillin, except for the introduction and use of serum antibodies and the discovery and use of salvarsan for the treatment of syphilis, physicians could do very little to help patients suffering from a serious infection. They could amputate a gangrenous leg or remove an inflamed appendix or gallbladder, but these problems occurred in only a few patients. Most of the time physicians simply waited for the patient's own immune system to overcome the infection; if this failed, the patient died. Such was the state of medical care of infections.

Let us return now to our story of the rediscovery of the same species of *Penicillium* by Alexander Fleming in September 1928.

Fleming was born in Lochfield, Scotland, in 1881. He was raised on a farm and attended the excellent schools for which Lowland Scots were famous during the Victorian era. A short, slim man, he chose two sports, swimming and rifle shooting, for his lifetime hobbies.[3]

After attending the University of London on a scholarship, he selected Saint Mary's Hospital for his medical school training because he had previously competed against Saint Mary's students in swimming and shooting contests. He graduated as a physician in 1906 on his twenty-fifth birthday. He was employed as an assistant in the inoculation department at Saint Mary's, not solely because of his medical school record, but also because his skill in shooting would strengthen the hospital's rifle team. He remained at Saint Mary's until he retired in 1955, dying three months later.

Fleming on entering the inoculation department at Saint Mary's became the assistant director, and he remained in that position until he retired. Sir Almroth Wright was the director when Fleming came into the department and was still the director when Fleming retired.

Almroth Wright was many things that Alexander Fleming was not. Wright was dictatorial and arrogant, Fleming was humble and shy; Wright was a forceful, colorful speaker, Fleming in the department was a colorless, boring lecturer. Wright disliked the administrative details of running the department, Fleming enjoyed such work. Wright was tall and patrician in aspect, Fleming was short and physically far from imposing. In short, whatever adjective one employed to describe Wright, one would use its antonym to describe Fleming. It was once said that when General George Marshall came through a door, those in the room immediately sensed that a presence had entered. When Fleming entered or left a meeting of his medical colleagues, none observed either his presence or his absence.

Strangely though, when he departed the laboratory, except for his short stature and slenderness he became a different person. He would stop regularly on his way home at the Chelsea Arts Club. There he met prominent London artists, many of whom had syphilis and were being treated by Fleming (one of the leading experts in the treatment of this dread disorder). A number of these artists gave him a painting in lieu of paying him for his services. In this unusual manner, Fleming gathered a large collection of paintings by some of the foremost London artists of his time.

In addition, he made so much money treating syphilitic patients that not only were he, his wife Amelia, and his children able to live in an opulent apartment in Chelsea, but he also acquired a large country mansion with its own stream and a huge garden. He tended the garden himself, growing vegetables for the family table, and frequently the family would dine on a fish that he had caught in his stream. Also, outside the laboratory he became positively gregarious, inviting guests to visit his country house or entertaining them at expensive London restaurants.

Just as spores of *Penicillium notatum* fell from the atmosphere into Tyndall's culture tubes a half-century before, so the same species of *Penicillium* entered by accident when Fleming opened one of his petri dishes to smear it with a strain of staphylococcus.

Tyndall exposed his broth cultures to the air of the room for twenty-four hours, so there was plenty of time for the few *Penicillium* spores present in the air to drop into his culture tubes and reproduce. Fleming, on the other hand, opened his petri dish for just a few seconds. Ordinarily this would have been too brief a time for a stray spore or two to find the dish. But on this occasion probably billions of *Penicillium* spores happened to be floating in the air of Fleming's laboratory, because one floor below his laboratory an expert on molds was growing *Penicillium notatum*. Since at that time there was no adequate method to stop spores from floating away, the spores, being very light, ascended the elevator shaft and the staircase to Fleming's laboratory door, which he habitually kept open.[4]

Because he was going on vacation for two weeks, he left the petri dish on his laboratory bench, ready to be placed in the incubator on his return. Lying on the bench, the staphylococci would multiply readily enough at room temperature; but they would have multiplied a billionfold in just twenty-four hours had they been placed in his incubator, which was set at body temperature.

On returning in September 1928 from his vacation, Fleming, again like Tyndall, noted that although a profuse growth of staphylococci occupied the surface of the agar culture plate, a wide area surrounding the circular growth of the *Penicillium* mold was devoid of staphylococci. Unlike Tyndall, Fleming decided to investigate this singular phenomenon.

He was almost unbelievably lucky in being able to rediscover the antibacterial capacity of the mold. A single change in the circumstances would have prevented this portentous rediscovery. For example, if he had inoculated the petri dish culture plate with some bacterium other than a staphylococcus that was immune to the antibacterial effect of *Penicillium* (of which there are many varieties), he would have observed no effect.

Fleming also was lucky in that the spores dropped into the petri dish at *precisely* the time that he smeared the agar culture with staphylococci. If the mold spores had found the petri dish hours after it had been inoculated and was already flourishing with staphylococci, the bacterial growth would have prevented multiplication of the *Penicillium* spores. This ability of bacterial colonies to inhibit the growth of *Penicillium notatum* was only discovered later.

Finally, Fleming was incredibly lucky in that he inoculated his petri dishes just before he went on a two-week vacation. It was usually his custom to put an inoculated petri dish in his incubator, but he knew that the staphylococci even at room temperature would multiply sufficiently for his purposes during the vacation period. There was no need to place the petri dishes in the incubator. What Fleming had no way of knowing was that the *Penicillium* mold grew as luxuriantly at room temperature as staphylococcus did in the 38° C of Fleming's incubator. At that incubator temperature, *Penicillium* does not grow at all. So if Fleming had not taken this particular vacation, he would have placed his petri dishes in the incubator, and next morning he would have obtained his expected luxuriant growth of staphylococci. But there would not have been the slightest trace of the mold spores that had accidentally entered the petri dish as he opened its cover to smear the plate with staphylococci. He would not have made the incredible discovery that led to the saving of millions of lives.

Fleming also was fortunate in that an intense heat wave hit London—so severe that the room temperature in his laboratory rose to the same temperature as that in his incubator. On the very day that he opened that petri dish and allowed the *Penicillium* spore to fall in, the heat wave broke. The temperature in his laboratory fell and remained low enough to allow the spore to grow during his vacation.

Fleming was too good a scientist to discard his mold-contaminated staphylococcus culture. When he saw that a wide, clear zone, totally devoid of staphylococci, surrounded the yellow-green growth of *Penicillium*, and that the rest of the culture plate was swarming with these same bacteria, he knew that he had made a discovery. And although he was preoccupied with his other laboratory studies, as well as his very lucrative private practice of shooting salvarsan into the veins of rich but syphilitic Londoners, he decided to look into the strange accident that greeted him on his return from vacation.

One of Fleming's first steps in this new study of a mold and its strange ability to stop the growth of staphylococci was to find out if the mold was able to inhibit the growth of any other bacteria. To accomplish this, Fleming had to contrive a suitable screening method. It did not take him long to ascertain that the broth upon whose surface the growing mold floated contained the substance that possessed antibacterial power. Fleming designated this still unknown substance *penicillin*. He found that, whatever it was, it was soluble and passed easily through a bacterial filter. He also observed that this penicillin only gradually accumulated in the broth upon whose surface the mold grew, reaching its maximum concentration in approximately eight days of mold growth.

The screening method Fleming devised was both simple and clever. He produced a narrow canal bisecting a round agar culture plate in a petri dish. Then he introduced into the canal a few drops of a mature mold broth containing penicillin. He brushed drops of various species of bacteria across the canal and along the agar culture plate, starting the streak of each drop of bacteria next to the canal and extending it to the periphery of the culture plate. Knowing that the penicillin in the broth he poured into the canal would diffuse somewhat outward into the agar culture plate, the species of bacteria sensitive to the penicillin would not grow near the canal.

Employing this method, Fleming found that most varieties of staphylococci, pneumococci, streptococci, gonococci, and meningococci did not grow near the canal containing the penicillin. These bacteria of course cause some of the deadliest of human infections. However effective this penicillin was against these species of bacteria, it still was virtually useless against other bacteria such as the bacilli that cause tuberculosis, influenza-like illnesses, and typhoid fever.

It seems almost unbelievable but Fleming—who was considered England's top therapist in the treatment of syphilis—never tested the effect of penicillin on the growth of the spirochete that causes this mightily dreaded disease. Had he done so, he would have found that his penicillin was overwhelmingly effective. As a matter of fact, syphilis can now be eradicated with penicillin or one of its derivatives in several weeks. When salvarsan was the method of treatment, it required weekly intravenous injections extending over a period of eighteen months.

Fleming examined other species of *Penicillium* to determine if one or more of them also possessed antibacterial potency, but he found no effective species other than the one that accidentally fell into his opened petri dish on that fateful September day in 1928. He injected the *Penicillium* broth filtrate into one rabbit and one mouse and determined that no ill results occurred. He even irrigated an infected human eye, an inflamed maxillary sinus, and the infected surface of an amputated leg with a penicillin solution. These three infected tissues not only showed no toxic effects from the penicillin, but all quickly lost their infection except for the patient whose leg had been amputated.

Given these observations of the astounding antibacterial efficacy of this accidentally discovered *Penicillium notatum*, why after publishing his first paper in 1929 and a trivial second report in 1932,[5] did Fleming give up his study of this amazing mold? There were a number of reasons.

Probably the most important was Fleming's odd inability to conceive of the possibility that a bacterial infection within the body could be helped by the injection or ingestion of a drug. Tragically, when he injected penicillin into one rabbit and a single mouse, he did not simultaneously inject either animal with a lethal strain of streptococci, staphylococci, or pneumococci. Had he done so, he would have been astonished by the survival of the animal despite the injection of such lethal bacteria.

This failure of Fleming to test the antibacterial power of his mold in an infected animal is partly understandable when we remember that his superior, Sir Almroth Wright, believed, as did all Fleming's colleagues, that "antibacterial drugs are a delusion."[6] But Wright cannot be entirely blamed for Fleming's failure to carry on his mold researches. Many years earlier, when Wright was given samples of the marvelous new antisyphilitic drug salvarsan by Paul Ehrlich, its synthesizer, he gave the samples to Fleming to try on syphilitic patients. Fleming thus became the first physician in England to treat syphilitic patients with this amazing drug.

It is puzzling, indeed almost incomprehensible, that Fleming, after decades of administering salvarsan by vein to scores of luetic patients and watching them overcome their loathsome disease, thought of penicillin only as a possible *external* germicide to apply to the surface of an infected wound. He never viewed it as a possible *chemotherapeutic* drug like salvarsan, which could be injected to combat serious systemic bacterial infections. When one reads Fleming's 1929 article and sees that he compares penicillin to carbolic acid, it becomes evident that the paradigm of Fleming's thoughts concerning the antibacterial action of penicillin was strictly limited to an externally applied wash or ointment. It was not the first time, nor would it be the last, that recognition of a revolutionary medical discovery was delayed for many years because medical thinking was constrained by an obsolete paradigm of reasoning.

It is only fair to Fleming to point out that in the 1940s, after penicillin's effectiveness in systemic bacterial infections had been generally accepted, he gave as his excuse for not continuing his penicillin research that he found that his preparations quickly lost their potency. If he had had the services of an expert biochemist, ways could have been found to extract penicillin from its broth and to store it indefinitely as a pure white crystal. But Wright would not tolerate the presence of a single experienced biochemist in the inoculation department because, he declared, "there is not enough of the humanist in chemists."

Further, Fleming, for six years before the fateful *Penicillium* contaminated his petri dish, had been preoccupied with an enzyme that he had isolated from the mucus of his own nose. The enzyme, which he named lysozyme, he believed might have antibacterial qualities. He became so intrigued with this trivial enzyme that he quit his work on penicillin to study the characteristics of lysozyme for the rest of his career.[7]

Although Fleming had deserted penicillin, his 1929 article describing its properties preserved it from oblivion. But a change in medical thinking needed to take place. Physicians had to begin to conceive, as Fleming had not, of the possibility that an injected or ingested drug might be effective in curing a systemic bacterial infection. A young bacteriologist named Paine, after reading Fleming's article, obtained from Fleming a sample of his *Penicillium notatum*, made broth cultures, then applied the mold to the infected eyes of four babies and the seriously injured and infected eye of an adult man. In forty-six hours this treatment dramatically cleared three of the four babies' eye infections as well as that of the man. Since two of the eye infections of the babies had been caused by gonococci, their eyesight would have been destroyed if their eyes had not been irrigated with what Dr. Paine called mold juice.

The bacteriologist was so excited about this curative effect of penicillin that he reported his results to none other than Howard Florey, at that time professor of pathology at Sheffield University.[8] This incident happened years before Florey began his own famous work with penicillin at Oxford. Apparently in the early 1930s Florey's mind, like Fleming's, was incapable of conceiving that a drug of any sort could cure a systemic bacterial infection.

Paine was not the only investigator in the early 1930s to read Fleming's article and decided to investigate further the properties of his penicillin. Harold Rainstrick, head of the newly established London School of Hygiene and Tropical Medicine, assembled an exceptionally strong team in 1931 to study the chemicals that various species of *Penicillium* produced. They asked Fleming for a sample of his mold, which he gladly sent. Rainstrick and his group in turn forwarded a sample of Fleming's mold to an American mycologist, who identified it as a variant form of *Penicillium notatum*. The Rainstrick group made the important observation that it was only Fleming's variant form, not the standard *Penicillium notatum*, that produced the antibacterial penicillin.[9]

How fortunate it was that this variant form of *Penicillium notatum* was the one that in 1928 floated into Fleming's petri dish. How fortunate it was also that Fleming continued to save this variant form, long after he had discontinued his own study of its antibacterial qualities. Unfortunately, when Rainstrick's group attempted to get a more concentrated strain by evaporating a solution of penicillin dissolved in ether, the penicillin became inactive. Because of this chemical failure, the London team stopped working with penicillin.

A young American graduate student in 1935 also began to study Fleming's *Penicillium notatum* and found that penicillin did not dissolve bacteria, but inhibited their growth. He wanted to continue his studies of penicillin and use his findings for his doctoral dissertation, but his supervising professor would not allow him to do so because he was sure that penicillin did not have any practical use. Nevertheless, R. D. Reid did describe his findings in a journal article.[10]

Perhaps the researches of Paine and Rainstrick would have been the last ever performed on penicillin if in 1935 Gerhard Domagk had not discovered that the injection of a simple compound, Prontosil, easily cured systemic streptococcal infections in man. This substance was synthesized in 1932 by a chemist working for I. G. Farbenindustrie of Germany in its search for new dyes. But the reddish Prontosil proved unsatisfactory as a practical dye and was set aside, along with scores of other dyes that were found unsatisfactory. Domagk, however, was not interested in finding new dyes to color clothes. As director of this company's department of pathology and bacteriology, he was interested in drugs that might kill bacteria.

When Domagk found that Prontosil, given intravenously, quickly cured patients of their streptococcal infection, he hastened to publish his results.[11] He thereby destroyed the stifling belief, so long held, that the injection of drugs was useless in combating bacterial infection. Indeed, if his article had been published in 1925 instead of 1935, Fleming would assuredly not have quit working on penicillin in 1928. Within several short years of the Prontosil publication, dozens of new drugs were investigated and found effective to combat certain systemic bacterial infections.

It was this new way of thinking that induced George Dreyer, professor and chairman of the Sir William Dunn School of Pathology at Oxford, after reading Fleming's 1929 paper, to resume the study of penicillin. Dreyer, one of the world's leading authorities on bacteriophages (viruses that infest and kill bacteria), had the hunch that penicillin also was a virus and that this property was responsible for its antibacterial action. So thinking, he asked for and obtained some of Fleming's *Penicillium notatum*. But when he tested this penicillin, he found it was not a virus.[12] Profoundly disappointed, he completely discontinued research on the mold and its product. However, instead of throwing away the mold, he allowed his assistant, a Miss Campbell-Renton, to continue growing it because she had found it extremely useful for other purposes. A few years later Dreyer died; Campbell-Renton kept the mold and allowed it to continue to survive.

Dreyer's successor at Oxford was a gifted Australian living in Britain. Howard Walter Florey, thirty-seven years old, was a physiologist, a pathologist, and a specialist in internal medicine. Florey married twice, both times to women who played significant roles in the utilization of penicillin. His first wife, Mary Ethyl Florey (later Lady Florey), was a physician who used penicillin for the treatment of infected wounds. By late 1942 she had already treated 172 patients successfully. Howard and Mary Ethyl met as fellow medical students at the University of Adelaide and married in 1926. She died in 1966; eight months later, Margaret Jennings, a collaborator on the famous paper by the Oxford team in 1940, became the second Lady Florey.

Howard Florey and the team he assembled at Oxford brought a new concept to the School of Pathology: instead of finding out what diseases or disease processes looked like, they decided to find out what was causing the pathology they could detect. Florey had great leadership qualities, a ready sense of humor, and a dedication to the task at hand—qualities that led him and his colleagues to make the first systematic discoveries regarding the true nature of penicillin.

Florey's team was in many ways as remarkable as its leader. Ernst Boris Chain, a talented musician as well as a biochemist, fled Nazi Germany to come to Britain, first to University College Hospital in London, and then to Cambridge. Just as Chain was deciding to take a new job in Australia, Florey persuaded him to join his new group at Oxford.

At Oxford Chain, who had (accidentally!) discovered Fleming's penicillin paper in the process of routine research, met Campbell-Renton in the corridor one day. She happened (again accidentally!) to be carrying a flask of Fleming's mold. Chain was surprised and delighted when he discovered what she had, because until that moment he had no idea that Oxford possessed any *Penicillium* whatsoever, to say nothing of some obtained from Fleming's own mold.

Chain went to Florey with a new idea. No one knew anything about the biochemical and biological properties of any antibacterial substances that microorganisms might possess. Chain was certain that there was a wonderful opportunity to do basic research in this area. Unlike Sir Almroth Wright, Florey was enthusiastic about this type of research.

But in 1939, as now, research required money. The School of Pathology had none for this purpose; nor did the British Medical Research Council. Undaunted, Florey asked the Rockefeller Foundation, with which he had previously been affiliated, what kinds of research projects they were prepared to support. The foundation's response was that it was not seeking projects intended to produce immediate practical results; it would be interested in funding proposals for research involving biochemistry, not clinical medicine. Chain and Florey were ecstatic; the projects they had in mind fit those criteria perfectly.

Once armed with Rockefeller Foundation funds, Chain and Florey went to work. They planned to generate not a clinically useful antibiotic for the war then being fought, but a body of fundamental research that might show how certain microorganisms produce, secrete, or otherwise elaborate antibacterial enzymes. This indeed was revolutionary thinking—searching for substances produced by one microorganism that might kill other microorganisms.

Chain's fortuitous encounter with Campbell-Renton of course made history. "We happened to go for penicillin," he later said, "because we had a culture growing at the school." [13] Neither he nor Florey had any idea that penicillin would turn out to be such a wonder drug.

Another outstanding scientist and member of the Oxford team, Margaret Jennings, found that penicillin had no effect on fully grown bacteria; its power lay in its ability to inhibit the growth of bacteria.

Norman Heatley, a painfully shy pioneer in microtechniques, joined the group when because of the war he could not study at the University of Copenhagen. It was Heatley who developed a method for determining the quantity of penicillin present in a given sample, and who defined a unit of penicillin activity. Without these determinations, physicians would not have been able to give penicillin to living patients.

Soon after the Oxford team began its work, Chain discovered that penicillin was not an enzyme but a simple molecule. Flabbergasted, surprised, and disappointed, he was on the point of closing down his research on penicillin, but its instability piqued his curiosity. For unlike other simple molecules, penicillin was exceedingly unstable. Chain finally overcame the problem by reducing the temperature of a water solution of penicillin by freeze-drying it. He produced, for the first time, a brown penicillin powder twenty times more potent than the most potent sulfa drug—and stable!

Was this new antibacterial substance safe? Amazingly, an enormous dose given to mice had no side effects. Chain knew enough about penicillin at this point to understand that he was on the threshold of one of the most far-reaching discoveries in the history of Western medicine. He told Florey what he had done. Like Chain, Florey was astounded; it seemed too good to be true. Florey repeated Chain's experiments himself, to be certain there was no mistake. Chain's results were indeed correct, and on this second experimental trial Chain and Florey noticed something else. After mice received the penicillin, their urine turned brown. Tests proved that the brown color was due to penicillin, which had passed unaltered, without loss of potency, into the urine.

The significance of this discovery was that penicillin could seep into fluids throughout the body. With this discovery Chain and Florey had produced what was probably the most powerful antibacterial substance known at that moment, which could probably be given safely by injection to humans. It could probably go anywhere in the body, making it possible to fight infections wherever they existed. It turned out, of course, that all these assumptions were correct; but Florey, Chain, and the Oxford team had a great deal of work to do before they could prove that their assumptions were correct.

The excitement at Oxford was intense — so intense, in fact, that Florey did something unheard of in Britain: he started an experiment on a Saturday. In British terms, the Oxford team was not simply excited; it almost came unhinged.

As it developed, Florey did what Fleming had failed to do: he experimented with penicillin on eight white mice. After injecting what should have been lethal doses of streptococci into the mice, he treated four with various doses of penicillin, leaving the other four untreated. The four mice who received penicillin all survived. The four who did not get penicillin did not survive. This tiny experiment on eight mice ushered in the era of antibiotics.

Heatley was so excited that he stayed up all night to see the outcome of the experiment. He was confronted (it was wartime) by a member of the Home Guard, concerned that he was breaking the curfew by riding his bicycle home in the small hours of a Sunday morning.

During the three months that followed this initial, never published pilot study, Florey and his group did extensive toxicity tests on animals, each of which demonstrated that penicillin had no harmful side effects. They also did five separate experiments, each involving forty-eight to seventy-five mice and using three different kinds of bacteria. In every case, the mice treated with penicillin lived, but only four of the untreated mice survived. These landmark experiments proved that, in mice, penicillin was by far the most effective chemotherapeutic agent produced to that point in time. The Oxford group published their remarkable results in a historic paper dated August 24, 1940.[14]

Only three months had elapsed between the initial pilot study and the publication of that first paper. The editors of *Lancet*, recognizing the landmark importance of the paper, gave it priority of publication. Those three months also were among the darkest hours of World War II. For this reason Florey, Chain, Heatley, and Jennings each rubbed penicillin mold on the inside of their clothing. If Germany should invade and occupy Britain, they hoped that one of them might escape to the United States or Canada with the spores of this mold, which they now knew might save far more lives than were being wasted by the war.

Shortly after they published their first paper, Florey's team repeated their animal experiments, with the same spectacular results. But at this point Florey reneged on his promise to the Rockefeller Foundation to investigate only the biochemistry of penicillin. The point had been to do pure scientific laboratory research, not to get bogged down in large-scale clinical studies. Britain, however, was at war, and infected wounds were — in this war as in all previous wars — the biggest killer. Florey knew that he had in his hands a chemotherapeutic agent that was potentially the most life-saving drug in the world. But it needed to be tested on patients, above all else, to prove whether this was indeed the case. Moreover, if further tests showed that the effects of penicillin were as miraculous as the initial results indicated, he would have to find a way to manufacture large quantities of it very rapidly to save as many lives as possible.

For the first test in human beings, Florey chose a patient with terminal cancer. Because gastric juices destroy penicillin, he gave the patient an intravenous drip; to his horror and dismay, the patient developed chills and a high fever. He knew immediately what this meant: that his penicillin mixture contained a toxic fever-producing impurity.

Much to the relief of the Oxford team, Abraham and Chain immediately set about to remove this toxic impurity. They succeeded and, to make the penicillin as pure as possible, they developed a complex, multistep extraction process that included subjecting the mixture twice to chromatography. The mixture needed to be made somewhat acid, and its temperature had to be kept at the freezing point to prevent the penicillin from being destroyed. This purification process later was beset with problems. In the end, the purified penicillin was freeze-dried, reducing it to a stable yellow powder.

Large-scale production of penicillin became an immediate problem in light of Florey's decision to conduct clinical trials on penicillin, rather than regard it as merely a topic of intellectual curiosity. Penicillin's potential was so great that he violated a long-established taboo: university departments are not to manufacture products, but are to be devoted to pure research. Sometimes only by breaking with tradition can individuals become "leaders." Florey certainly did so when he established the so-called production department, a minifactory within his academic department at Oxford.

Heatley took the first step when he improved the medium on which the mold was cultured. He then devised a unique way to collect the mold juice. In the conventional method, each mold colony could only be used once and then it broke up. Heatley prevented this from happening by blowing air under the well-developed mold colony so as to keep it elevated and intact. He then withdrew the mold juice and replaced it with fresh culture medium. Using this method, he obtained twelve samples of mold juice from each culture. (Later he developed an automatic extraction plant that increased even this output.)

One process Heatley could not automate, however. Since the newly established purification process involved reducing the temperature of the penicillin mixture to the freezing point, then rolling the glass bottles containing the mixture, a basic problem resulted: there were not enough hands to do the rolling. No additional male hands were available, because men who might otherwise have been recruited were serving in the armed services. But hands are hands, male or female. Breaking another taboo, the group for the first time in Oxford history hired a small number of women who, eight hours a day, rolled bottles of penicillin back and forth in a freezing room. They became known as the penicillin girls.

At this point Heatley simply ran out of room. He thought he could solve the problem by using shallow, flat, oblong culture dishes that occupied less space than glass bottles; but the manufacturers of those dishes said they could not make any for at least six months, and then at a price so outrageously high that the department could not afford to purchase them. Florey, ever the problem-solving entrepreneur, contacted a physician whom he knew at Stoke-on-Trent, the pottery capital of the world. Informed of the problem, the friend asked Florey to send him a sketch of what was wanted. The physician found a local firm willing to manufacture dishes rapidly, and for a reasonable price. Heatley visited the pottery, selected one of three prototype dishes, and within a few weeks had as many as he could use.

A year later, Florey found a novel way to expand his production department. The university pathology department had an animal postmortem house, which was not unusual. What was unique was that the house had been built specifically for performing postmortem studies on rhinoceroses and elephants. Thus it was large enough and convenient enough to become Florey's first penicillin "factory."

Meantime, the study of penicillin in human patients was progressing rapidly. Florey and his colleagues had injected penicillin intravenously into everyone at the Sir William Dunn Department of Pathology, without ill effects. Before the group had accumulated enough penicillin to start wide-scale testing in human beings, Florey was asked to treat a desperately ill policeman dying of septicemia. At first the treated patient improved dramatically, but he required such high doses of penicillin Florey's supply was depleted. He and his colleagues tried to reclaim some of the penicillin from the patient's urine, but even with this desperate step they ran out. The policeman became hopelessly ill again and died. Florey vowed never again to treat a patient unless a sufficient supply of penicillin was on hand.

Once again, Florey hit on a unique solution to test penicillin in human beings, even though the available supply was small. The supply was small? Then let us, Florey reasoned, treat small patients. The first studies accordingly involved very young children. Four suitable candidates were located, plus a fifth subject who was a small adult. The results were amazing. All the children were cured, save one who had an infected blood clot in a vein at the base of his skull, adjacent to which lay the carotid artery. The walls of the artery had also become infected, causing it to balloon out and form an aneurysm. Although the infection subsided, the aneurysm ruptured and the patient died from a massive brain hemorrhage. (An autopsy confirmed that penicillin had completely cured the infection.) The Oxford team was amazed at the striking clinical results. Florey, who always couched his descriptions in the most cautious terms, remarked that the outcome in these patients was "almost miraculous." The results were published in August 1941.[15]

Shortly thereafter, Chain wanted to patent penicillin. Florey did not agree, believing that it was unethical to do so. Florey and Chain had many heated debates on the issue, but Florey held firm. Chain feared that if the Oxford group did not obtain a patent, others would; as it later developed, he was right.

Realizing that the so-called production department at Oxford could never meet Britain's wartime need for penicillin, Florey spoke to the executives of every pharmaceutical company in Britain, urging them to manufacture penicillin. Imperial Chemical Industries did begin the requisite experiments, but talks with other companies were unavailing.

Florey, having received additional penicillin from Imperial Chemical Industries, gave penicillin to 15 patients intravenously and to 172 patients locally, beginning in January 1942. By measuring the blood levels of penicillin and studying its clinical effects, he established the appropriate dosage for each condition treated. No government agency today would allow any drug given intravenously to be generally distributed after it had been tried on only twenty-one patients, two of whom had died; nor would it allow any drug to be distributed if, like penicillin, it killed guinea pigs. But Florey's meticulous observations, made under exceedingly difficult wartime conditions, proved convincing enough. And luckily Florey did not include guinea pigs among his test animals.

At about this time Sir Almroth Wright wrote a famous letter to the *London Times* in which he named Fleming as penicillin's discoverer. The editor, Robert Robertson, responded by naming Florey. The result, no surprise in today's era of media saturation, was that hordes of reporters descended on both Fleming and Florey. Incredibly, though, both men underwent a personality transformation: Fleming now sought publicity, Florey sought privacy. No one has ever been able to explain this reversal.

In any case, newspapers report what people are willing to tell them. Since Fleming would talk and Florey would not, the newspapers were filled with news about Fleming and almost nothing about Florey. Most of the stories were exaggerated and untrue, but Fleming made no attempt to correct them. Even medical journals and books began to publish pure fiction about the history of penicillin, based on the newspaper reports. Fleming laughed at what the news media said about him, joked about the media viewpoint to his friends, and had his secretary file all erroneous press clippings and journal articles.

All of this lightheartedness had consequences. Years later Lord Beaverbrook, the newspaper owner, who had obtained a one-sided and erroneous view of the history of penicillin from his reporters and who may have felt that Florey had snubbed him, urged the Nobel committee to award its Prize in Physiology or Medicine to Fleming alone.

After reading the Oxford group's 1941 paper in the *Lancet*, Fleming decided to see for himself what these scientists were doing. Chain had the honor of giving the visitor the grand tour of the department. Fleming was his former introverted self, never uttering a word and leaving Chain with the impression that Fleming had not understood anything that was shown him.

Shortly thereafter, Fleming asked Florey for some penicillin to treat a patient on the verge of death. Florey, whose stock of penicillin was almost gone, agreed on condition that he be allowed to include the patient in his current clinical series. After receiving the penicillin, Fleming's patient made an extraordinary recovery. It impressed Fleming so much that he contacted a close friend, Sir Andrew Duncan, the British minister of supply, to request government aid in producing penicillin.

During the early part of the war, Britain had successfully evacuated its troops from the beach at Dunkirk by means of a large number of small (mainly private) sailing vessels, scattered widely so that it was impossible for the Luftwaffe to bomb them all. Thinking along similar lines, the British penicillin committee decided not to build a single, large, central plant, which the Germans could easily destroy. Rather, penicillin was produced in every conceivable kind of facility, using whatever equipment was available. Milk cans and bottles—in fact, any bottles at all—were used to culture the mold. Although a few fairly large companies manufactured penicillin in commercial quantities, a "mom and pop" industry evolved, in which basement laboratories all over Britain worked to produce penicillin in the necessary quantities. Penicillin from every source was then pooled. The Ministry of Supply furnished precious gasoline for the vehicles needed to transport the penicillin (as well as other items in short supply during wartime, including tin cans). Amazingly, in this manner Britain produced all the penicillin necessary for its armed forces and its civilian population during World War II.

One of Florey's best and most consistent sources of penicillin was a company called Kendall, Bishop. Its factory was in East London. Because many industries and dockyards were also located there, the East End became a prime target for German bombers. Every building in the blocks surrounding Kendall, Bishop was destroyed, but somehow the nation's best and most consistent industrial source of penicillin stood, unharmed, amid the surrounding rubble.

Shortly after the Oxford team's first paper in 1940, American physicians and researchers began to make major contributions as well. Indeed, the first patient treated systemically with penicillin was not at Oxford, but at Columbia Presbyterian Hospital in New York. His physician, Dr. Martin Henry Dawson, assembled a small but outstanding team, consisting of himself, Dr. Karl Meyer, a biochemical genius who many believed deserved the Nobel Prize, and Dr. Gladys Hobby, an outstanding microbiologist and the author of a book on the history of penicillin.[16] Five weeks after the Oxford team's first paper appeared in the *Lancet*, this American group started treating patients, using mold provided by Dr. Roger Reed. (Chain had sent a batch of *Penicillium*, but that specimen produced no penicillin.) Dawson's group presented its results at a meeting of the American Society for Clinical Investigation in May 1941.

Howard Florey's visit to the United States and Canada that same year, however, provided the strongest impetus to the further production and clinical use of penicillin in North America. Several factors convinced Florey to undertake this historic trip. First, he heard that the Germans had attempted to find out about penicillin through the Swiss, so he warned everyone who might have the mold not to give a sample to any foreigner. Second, he trusted the North Americans and felt that they would support Britain in the war. Third, with the sole exception of Imperial Chemical Industries, all the British pharmaceutical companies had rejected his overtures to manufacture penicillin. Finally, Sir Edward Mellanby, secretary of the British Medical Research Council, who had vigorously recommended Florey's appointment at Oxford, suggested that he go to the United States and Canada to get the vast economic and manufacturing potential of North America behind the full-scale production of penicillin. Florey managed to obtain funding for the trip from the Rockefeller Foundation and took a sample of the mold with him.

Florey, with Norman Heatley, arrived in New York on July 3, 1941, and on Independence Day were entertained by Professor John Fulton and his wife in New Haven. Fulton later arranged for the two men to visit Dr. Robert Coghill, who headed the fermentation division of the U.S. Department of Agriculture's Northern Regional Research Laboratory at Peoria, Illinois. Coghill welcomed the pair warmly, offering his full support. During their conversation he suggested that deep fermentation—a process that involved submerging the mold beneath the surface of the culture medium, possibly making the production of penicillin more efficient and convenient—might be the ideal method of production. In this he was correct. Deep fermentation would be the single most important contribution of the United States to the mass production of penicillin.

Coghill arranged for Heatley to work with Dr. Andrew Moyer, a biochemist on the Peoria staff. Moyer was a rogue and rabidly anti-British. An agreement was signed by the Rockefeller Foundation, which gave financial support to Heatley, and the Northern Regional Research Laboratory, which supported Moyer, that the pair should publish all their work jointly, and that the foundation and the laboratory should share all royalties derived from patents. Heatley taught Moyer everything he knew about penicillin. Moyer, in turn, came up with the idea of adding corn-steep liquor and lactose, highly nutritious substrates for molds, to the culture medium, thereby increasing the production of penicillin twenty-fold.

Before Heatley left the United States, he and Moyer wrote a paper on their work. They met to discuss the final draft and Moyer agreed with all of Heatley's changes. But after Heatley left, Moyer deleted Heatley's name from the paper and published it on his own. As sole author, Moyer was entitled to patent the use of corn-steep liquor and lactose for growing penicillin molds. Although the foundation and the laboratory would have to share all royalties from patents awarded in the United States, Moyer discovered a loophole and filed for three patents in Britain. He did not reap the riches his treachery may have led him to expect; for justice did prevail. Under pressure from Coghill, the Department of Agriculture forced Moyer to return every cent he earned to the two backers.

Eventually both U.S. and British pharmaceutical companies filed for other patents—in the United States for deep fermentation, and in Britain for semisynthetic penicillins. To avoid bankrupting their financially strapped British allies, the American companies asked the lowest possible royalties and even reduced those charges several times. Still, the royalties British pharmaceutical companies had to pay their American counterparts cost millions of dollars, losses recouped only later when semisynthetic penicillins became available.

While all of these maneuverings were going on, Dr. Kenneth B. Raper, the mycologist at Peoria, was scouring the world for better examples of penicillin-producing *Penicillium*. The best specimen turned up in his own backyard. Raper had assigned one of his assistants to bring back all the fruit she could find at the local market, and subsequently managed to isolate *Penicillium chrysogenum* from a cantaloupe she had purchased. It produced more penicillin than any other mold in the world and grew beautifully in the culture medium during deep fermentation. His famous assistant was called Moldy Mary for the rest of her life.

After Florey returned to Britain, several events soured his very cordial relationship with his American colleagues. After the United States entered the war in December 1941, the Americans steadfastly refused to disclose any information about the experimental work they were doing with penicillin, claiming it was a wartime secret—this despite Heatley's having given the Americans full details of the work done at Oxford. As it turned out, the deep-fermentation production technique discovered by American scientists would have allowed the British to increase their output of penicillin much sooner than they did. At the first meeting of the penicillin committee in Britain, Florey expressed his outrage at the American behavior in no uncertain terms. Members of the committee, impressed by Florey's testimony, initiated negotiations with their American counterparts that helped to resolve the problem.

Later, when news of the American patents broke, Florey was again angry; in fact, the matter remained a sore point between Chain and Florey throughout their lives. After the war the disgruntled Chain left Oxford, worked for a time in Italy, but returned to Britain to assume the post of professor and chairman of the department of biochemistry at the Imperial College of Science and Technology in London.

Other points of contention cropped up. The American Gladys Hobby claimed that penicillin was not the first antibiotic used in the treatment of infections in humans, that instead it was René Dubos' gramicidin.[17] This antibiotic is applied locally to treat infections and is currently mixed with two other antibiotics in the form of eyedrops to treat eye infections. Years earlier, though, Fleming and Paine had treated eye infections with so-called mold juice; and, most important, penicillin could be injected, given systemically, whereas gramicidin could not.

Coghill in Peoria had the brilliant idea of developing genetic mutations of Raper's cantaloupe mold that would produce more penicillin. He asked leading scientists around the country to try to do this by subjecting specimens of Raper's mold to light, to X rays, or to chemicals. Scientists at the Carnegie Institute at Cold Spring Harbor, New York, by irradiating *Penicillium chrysogenum* with X rays, succeeded in producing a mutant that yielded ten times more penicillin than the original mold had done.

Penicillin research in the United States was supervised by the Office of Scientific Research and Development. That office conducted highly successful clinical trials on the value of penicillin in treating bacterial pneumonia, chronic bone infections, wound infections, infections of the heart valves, gonorrhea, and syphilis. Hearing the results of these trials, three American pharmaceutical companies (Squibb, Merck, and Pfizer) became interested in producing penicillin, and Squibb and Merck instituted a collaborative program. Subsequently the Office of Scientific Research and Development selected twenty-two companies to manufacture penicillin in the United States, each of which was granted preferential treatment in construction materials and supplies during the first half of World War II.

Fleming, Florey, Chain, and Abraham received many honors and awards for their outstanding contributions to medicine. Fleming and Florey were knighted in 1944. The Nobel Prize in Physiology or Medicine was awarded to Fleming, Florey, and Chain in 1945. Chain and Abraham were knighted in 1965 and 1980, respectively. And Fleming received Britain's highest posthumous honor: on March 11, 1955, he was buried in the crypt of Saint Paul's Cathedral in London. Shortly thereafter, the inoculation department at Saint Mary's Hospital was renamed the Wright-Fleming Institute.

Penicillin has forever changed the treatment of infections. Once initial development efforts had succeeded, semisynthetic penicillins, and penicillins that can be taken by mouth were developed. More powerful antibiotics soon followed. The first was streptomycin, a broad-spectrum antibiotic developed by Selman A. Waksman and his colleagues at Rutgers University.[18] (Waksman was the person who had coined the term *antibiotic*.) Streptomycin was of particular importance because it was effective in treating tuberculosis and certain other bacterial infections that were not helped by penicillin.

Shortly thereafter, pharmaceutical companies announced other broad-spectrum antibiotics: Lederle Laboratories came up with Aureomycin in 1948, and Pfizer announced Terramycin in 1950. The first entirely synthetic antibiotic, Chloramphenicol, was developed by Parke-Davis in 1949 and proved particularly effective in the treatment of typhoid fever. Thus, Fleming's observation in 1929 had by midcentury spawned a huge pharmaceutical industry manufacturing a vast array of antibiotics. Contemporary investigators in the U.S. pharmaceutical industry, however, have become far more cautious, aware that it might cost more than $200 million to bring *any* new drug to the market, so exacting have become the approval criteria of the Food and Drug Administration.

Another problem is that bacteria are becoming resistant to the drugs we use to attack them, including penicillin. The percentage of pneumococcal strains, for example, that are drug resistant has risen from 0.02 percent in 1987 to 6.6 percent in 1994. In our supposed chemotherapeutic era, the unbelievable fact is that the cause of death in 13,300 hospital patients in the United States in 1994 was drug-resistant bacterial infections.[19]

Five decades ago, physicians believed that with the advent of streptomycin, tuberculosis would by 2000 have become as extinct as smallpox is. But the genes of certain strains of the tubercle bacillus somehow found ways to resist the usual antibacterial action of streptomycin. As a consequence of the emergence of these resistant strains, eight million humans a year become seriously infected with tuberculosis, and despite all chemotherapeutic efforts two million of them die.

Doctors themselves are to blame for some cases of drug-resistant bacterial infections, because too often they are tempted to treat viral infections with antibiotics in order to give the patient the impression that they are doing something (despite the fact that these doctors know that many viral infections are not susceptible to antibiotics).

The answer might seem simple: develop antibiotics that are effective against these new mutant strains of bacteria. Dr. Barry R. Bloom, a national leader in tuberculosis research at the Albert Einstein School of Medicine, and his colleagues Dr. William Jacobs and Dr. James Sachettni, have developed six new experimental drugs that were effective in vitro against drug-resistant tubercle bacilli; but no drug company thus far has chosen to develop them.[20] As we have pointed out, it can cost more than $200 million to get the government's permission to introduce a new drug. This economic factor is not forgotten for one instant by the head of any pharmaceutical company. Moreover, even after a drug is approved, its use may be catastrophically stopped by a side effect that does not become evident for years. Such has been the disastrous fate of more than one new drug in the past decade.

Despite the outrageous expense associated with the introduction of a new antibiotic drug, pharmaceutical companies will continue to search for promising new antibiotics and other sorts of drugs that may be of help in combating viruses and parasites that still are not affected by our present antibiotics.

IO

Maurice Wilkins and DNA

We had not been with eighty-three-year-old Erwin Chargaff, emeritus professor of biochemistry at Columbia University, for more than several minutes before he pointed to the 1871 volume of a bound set of German medical journals lying on one of his bookshelves. He cried out in Viennese-accented English, "You want to know who really deserves the major credit for the DNA discovery?" Without waiting for a response, he continued, "It's Friedrich Miescher, and he described his discovery in this 1871 article." [1] Chargaff's index finger continued to point to the bound volume.

"We're afraid we've never heard of him," we meekly commented.

"No, I was sure of that, but you've heard of James Watson and Francis Crick, Nobel laureates, our mass-media substitutes for saints."

"We've also heard of Maurice Wilkins, Rosalind Franklin, Oswald

Avery, Fred Griffith, and Max von Laue," we replied defensively and perhaps a bit angrily.

"Miescher discovered DNA as a chemical entity. Isn't that important to you?"

"Yes, very important; we shall look him up when we return to San Francisco." And we did.

Chargaff was correct, and we begin this account with a description of Friedrich Miescher's great discovery, even though he received only single-sentence or footnote recognition in any English scientific and medical publication until the famous 1953 articles on deoxyribonucleic acid (DNA) appeared in *Nature.* Three books briefly describing the work of Miescher were published in the 1970s.[2]

Miescher, a German-speaking Swiss, began his research in 1868 at Tübingen, in the laboratory of the illustrious biochemist Ernst Hoppe-Seyler. Miescher was shy and rather reticent, but he knew the question he wanted to answer: which chemicals made up the nucleus of a cell?

Prior to Miescher's studies, no one knew what the nucleus of a cell did, much less of what it was composed. Not only were pure suspensions of cells hard to obtain, but it was also difficult to separate or extract the tiny, microscopic nuclei from the cytoplasm of the cells in which they were embedded.

Miescher overcame both difficulties. Remembering that the white cells of blood contained relatively large nuclei and not much cytoplasm, he decided to collect such cells. But where could they be obtained? Miescher found a filthy answer: he collected the surgical bandages discarded by a Tübingen clinic. Swarming with white blood cells in the form of pus, these bandages furnished him with a dreadful, nauseating source of nucleated cells.

Mostly by repeated chemical trial and error, he was able to separate the nuclear material from the cytoplasm of these human pus cells. The chemical substance that he finally extracted and purified, he called *nuclein.* Although he knew that this nuclein contained protein, he recognized that an additional, heretofore unknown chemical substance was attached to the protein component. Because this new substance was so rich in phosphorus, Miescher hypothesized that nuclein served as the nucleus' way of continuously supplying phosphorus to the cell's cytoplasm. Even at age twenty-four or twenty-five, Miescher knew that he had made an awesome discovery; but his chief, Hoppe-Seyler, refused to release his paper in 1869. He delayed publication for two years until he himself could verify its accuracy. Today a bright young investigator so thwarted in publishing an article that he believed to be of prime importance probably would consult an attorney or complain to the Office of Scientific Integrity of the National Institutes of Health. But Miescher requested only that when his article was finally published in 1871, it bear a note indicating that it had been ready in 1869, to protect the priority of his magnificent discovery.

Miescher was aware that this newly discovered nucleoprotein had a high molecular weight. In a truly prescient comment, he pointed out that a compound as large and complex as nuclein might possibly function as a genetic substance. In a letter to his uncle in 1892, he wrote that his nuclein was a very large and complex molecule and that the isomerism of its carbon atoms alone could furnish a sufficient number of differently acting molecules to carry the myriad genetic characteristics. In an extraordinarily apt analogy, he pointed out that such chemical transmission might be similar to the fact that all the words and concepts of any language "can find expression" by the use of twenty to thirty alphabetic letters of that language. He was correct, for Shakespeare employed approximately thirty-five thousand different words in his plays and poems—but the twenty-six letters of our alphabet made up that profusion of words.

Yet no one took notice of this first hint of a hereditary code for fifty-one years. Then, in 1943, Erwin Schrödinger introduced the concept of genetic coding.

Forward looking as Miescher might have been in his concept of hereditary transmission, he did not suspect that it was only the nucleic acid component of his nuclein that might serve as the hereditary material. Like those who followed him for half a century, he believed that it was the protein component that served as the possible transmitter of heredity.

Miescher left Hoppe-Seyler's laboratory in 1871, either before or shortly after the publication of his discovery in Hoppe-Seyler's own journal, to assume the chair in physiology at Basel. There he remained until his death in 1895.

During this twenty-four-year tenure, he occupied himself mostly with teaching and constructing Switzerland's first Institute for Anatomical and Physiological Research. This building, the Vesalianum, still stands. At the top of its flight of steps, almost hidden from view, is a small bust of Miescher. As far as we know, this bust and the 1871 paper (the one that Chargaff pointed to during our 1988 visit with him) are the only tangible bits of evidence that this remarkable man once existed. But a few months before he died, he received a letter from Carl Ludwig, Europe's renowned physiologist, assuring the dying man that he would be remembered forever.

Miescher did learn before his death that his colleague Richard Altmann had been able in 1889 to free nuclein of its protein component, and had called what remained nucleic acid. He probably also became aware of the fact that Albrecht Kossel, the German biochemist, found that nuclein contained purines and pyrimidines. The exact number of these bases, however, was not determined. Kossel received a Nobel Prize in 1910, as did Altmann in 1912, for their other remarkable biochemical achievements.

Although it was suspected before the turn of the century that nucleic acids contained phosphate, purine, and pyrimidine molecules, it was not until 1909 that the gifted but erratic biochemist Phoebus A. Levene discovered a sugar in yeast nucleic acid—D-ribose. Twenty years later he detected a different sugar, 2-deoxy-D-ribose, in thymus nucleic acid.

Levene, like Miescher, believed that nucleic acids were very large macromolecular complexes consisting of what he designated as *nucleotides* (units consisting of phosphate, sugar, and purine/pyrimidine bases). Despite these significant contributions, he still believed that the hereditary-bearing substance in the nucleus dwelled in its proteins. And he could not conceive that such a simple macromolecule, composed of just a sugar, a phosphate, several purines and pyrimidines, and some water molecules, could send the billion or more macro and micro hereditary instructions that human chromosomes were known to transmit.

Both Miescher and Levene were well aware, since the epochal discoveries of Louis Pasteur and others, that the properties of a *molecule* were dependent not just on its atomic constituents but also on the physico-chemical interrelationships of these same atoms. They were not aware, nor were any of their contemporaries, that the properties of a *macromolecule* also were not just dependent on its molecular components but also on the interrelationships of these components. New discoveries, and touches of genius, would be required before chemists and biologists of the twentieth century stumbled on the fact that just as a mere twenty-six letters of the English alphabet permit the formation of vast numbers of different words, so the relatively few different molecules of the macromolecule DNA, by their myriad possible combinations, provide this seemingly simple macromolecule with the means of carrying billions of hereditary messages.

In 1912 the German physicist Max von Laue made a discovery that Einstein described as one of the most beautiful in all physics. He observed that exposure of a simple crystal to X-rays resulted in the registration of specific shadows on a photographic plate. Very soon after von Laue's announcement, these shadows were found by William Bragg to arise from diffraction of the original X-rays by their collision with the atoms in a crystal. Subsequently Bragg together with his son, William Lawrence Bragg, observed that the spots made on photographic films by X-rays traversing crystals were not only specific for each crystal but also yielded, on adequate study, an understanding of the spatial structure of the atoms making up any crystal. Through their invention of the science and art of crystallography, it was now possible to determine the atomic architecture of any crystal.

Decades later, scientists would develop the crystallographic expertise to determine the *intermolecular* relationships of macromolecules such as nucleic acid. Also, other advances had to occur before nucleic acid intrigued scientists sufficiently for them to investigate its suspension of purines, pyrimidines, sugars, and phosphates.

In 1927 Fred Griffith, a British physician, observed an extraordinarily puzzling event. When he injected mice subcutaneously with a culture of living but harmless pneumococci—plus a killed species of deadly pneumococci—the mice died the next day, and their death was caused by offspring of the previously harmless strain of pneumococci. These pneumococcal progeny had been changed into the same deadly species that the day before had killed prior to injection. Even more mysterious, these once harmless but now deadly bacteria continued to impart these identical deadlines to their progeny—forever!

How in the totally commonsensical world of science could the dead give rise to this sort of living miracle? Not for a split second did Griffith or his contemporaries (who confirmed his finding) ever suspect that the substance extracted from human pus by Miescher forty years earlier was responsible for this lethal transformation of a strain of harmless pneumococci.

Griffith probably had never heard of Miescher, nor perhaps of DNA. So he concluded that the killed culture of toxic pneumococci furnished the living and thriving avirulent pneumococci with what he described as a "pabulum," whose ingestion somehow caused the avirulent pneumococci to give rise to virulent ones. He was so convinced of this theory that he quite overlooked the fact that the virulent offspring of the initially avirulent species succeeded generation after generation in passing on their deadly virulence, in the complete absence of his pabulum.[3]

Despite this erroneous conclusion concerning the mechanism responsible for the observed bacterial transformation, Griffith's discovery was of monumental importance. Of course, it did not attract any interest at all from the geneticists, who were still totally absorbed in the genetics of their favorite experimental object, the common fruit fly. Griffith's epochal observations did in 1931 catch the skeptical attention of a very shy, short, balding bachelor, Oswald Theodore Avery, a Canadian-born physician-turned-scientist working at the Rockefeller Institute.

Avery, as a young man working with his biochemist colleague Michael Heidelberger, discovered the chemical nature of the capsular coverings of the four types of pneumococci, which not only were responsible for their toxicity but also for their serological specificity. The two men also found that the capsule of each type of pneumococcus was composed of a specific polysaccharide.

The four polysaccharides, although made up of similar, simple sugar molecules, differed markedly from one another in their biological properties. It is probable that this finding alerted Avery early in his career that the biological properties of any *macromolecule* depend on the interrelationships of its molecules. This was not a fact well recognized by even the most distinguished biochemists until the second half of this century. Indeed, if Miescher or his immediate successors had been aware of the dependence of a macromolecule for its biological properties on the interrelationships of its constituent molecules, the hereditary function of DNA would not have had to wait for over a half-century for its recognition. This new and fruitful truth might not have been completely obvious to Avery even in 1930, when he decided to have his subordinates determine if there were any truth in Griffith's bewildering discovery.

It was not very long before Avery's assistants confirmed Griffith's findings. J. Lionel Alloway reported that he was able to transform nonvirulent to virulent pneumococci simply by adding an extract of dead virulent pneumococci to a colony of nonvirulent pneumococci growing in a test tube. Avery then became enthusiastically and indefatigably committed to determining the nature of the substance that was transforming the pneumococcus from one type to another. Nor did his fulminating hyperthyroidism, which almost incapacitated him for four years, subvert his dogged determination to identify this chemical. When Griffith was killed in 1941 by a German bomb, Avery obtained a photograph of him, which remained on his desk until he retired from the Rockefeller Institute.

Avery did not work alone. Colin MacLeod, also a Canadian physician, joined him in 1935 and Maclyn McCarty, a newly graduated Johns Hopkins physician, in 1941. Both physicians contributed immensely to the thirteen-year search for the chemical identity of what they called the transforming principle.

Early in their analyses of the extracts of transforming principle, they detected a moderate amount of DNA. Although traces of other chemicals were present, including moderate amounts of protein, it was the genius of one or more members of the Avery-MacLeod-McCarty team to choose the DNA fraction as the object of intense investigation. We shall never be certain of the identity of this person or persons. But we can be sure that as the team's leader, if Avery did not make this analytical decision, at least he had to agree with it.

For years, then, these three physicians employed every immunological, chemical, biological, and physicochemical tool available to isolate DNA, and only DNA, from specific extracts. Early on, when they tested any DNA isolate of an extract, it possessed the transforming principle. The difficulty came in ridding the DNA completely of any trace of the protein with which it had been conjoined as the nucleoprotein component of the pneumococcus. No one recognized better than Avery the almost universal belief that only a protein, with its known complexity, could serve as the transforming principle. He remembered only too well his earlier difficulty in getting his colleagues to accept the truth that the toxin in the capsule of a pneumococcus was due to a complex sugar, not a protein.

Perhaps the most dramatic demonstration of the transforming capability of DNA was the specific loss of this capacity when a serum enzyme known to destroy DNA was added. Several years later, chiefly because of McCarty's efforts, the team reported the successful isolation and purification of this DNA-destroying enzyme.

On December 10, 1943, at the strong urging of his associates, in a lecture to all his Rockefeller Institute colleagues, Avery announced that pure DNA obtained from killed Type III encapsulated pneumococci was capable of transforming a culture of unencapsulated Type II pneumococci into Type III encapsulated pneumococci.

At the conclusion of the talk, according to McCarty,[4] his colleagues applauded Avery; but when the chairman called for questions or comments, a dead and embarrassing silence fell. Finally, one of Avery's former colleagues rose and described the many years that had gone into the study whose results had just been presented. He sat down. Dr. Schneider, the chairman, later reported to McCarty: "Another long silence ensued. At last, when I could stand it no longer, I said, 'This company, having reached unanimity of opinion, is now adjourned.'"

The key publication demonstrating DNA as the chemical substance responsible for the transforming principle appeared in the February 1944 issue of the *Journal of Experimental Medicine.*[5]

As McCarty told us in our 1990 conversation with him, the immediate reactions to their article were hardly breathtaking. Few if any geneticists ever read the *Journal of Experimental Medicine.* Also, in wartime 1944, the *New York Times* and any news magazine had too many more dazzling stories to report than an account of how an arcane chemical such as DNA could transform a Type III pneumococcus to Type II.

Far more damaging to acceptance of their paper was the obdurate refusal of Alfred Mirsky, a first-rate biochemist and fellow member of the Rockefeller Institute, to accept DNA as the carrier of the transforming principle. Apparently he could not believe that DNA, composed as it was of only several purines and pyrimidines, some phosphates, and sugars, could serve in this capacity. Only a complex protein was capable of carrying so many messages.

He spoke inside and outside the halls of the institute against the DNA concept proposed by Avery and his colleagues. Indeed, in a lecture in April 1946 to essentially the same Rockefeller Institute members to whom Avery had presented his DNA concept, Mirsky mercilessly attacked the Avery team's conclusions. Despite the group's meticulous elimination of any possible protein residue, Mirsky insisted that their supposedly pure DNA solution still might contain 1 to 2 percent protein, a quantity quite sufficient to act as carrier of the transforming principle.

Avery sat in the audience listening to this blistering attack. At no time did he attempt to refute Mirsky's indictment; he remained completely silent. Nor did Avery attempt to contradict Mirsky's published denial of the DNA role in carrying the transforming principle. But he became severely depressed in 1946 and accomplished little in the years between the 1944 announcement of DNA's role and his quiet retirement in 1948. Just as William Harvey had done three centuries earlier, Oswald Avery, now seventy-one tired years old, left the world of science to live obscurely but peacefully for the remaining seven years of his life with his brother Roy in Nashville, Tennessee.

He probably was disappointed that the discovery of DNA as the hereditary substance was neither recognized nor appreciated as one of the century's most momentous events. He probably did not know that he was nominated in the late 1940s for the Nobel Prize, but because of Mirsky's stubborn failure to acknowledge the validity of Avery's DNA conclusions, the Nobel committee thought it wise to postpone the award and await further confirmation of his discovery.

We shall never know how Avery felt when in 1953 he read the findings of Wilkins, Watson, Crick, and Franklin. Certainly his colleague Colin Mac-Leod was far from impressed by their discovery of the structure of DNA. We say this because McCarty gave us a copy of a note sent to him by MacLeod after he had read Watson's *Double Helix*. His note reads:

Some day perhaps you will enlighten me about the earthshaking significance of the double helix, etc. If it hadn't been worked out on a Tuesday, it would have happened in some other laboratory on Wednesday or Thursday.

Yours in frustration,
Colin

Obviously MacLeod and also Maclyn McCarty were more than a little disappointed that their disclosure concerning the hereditary potential of DNA received so little immediate attention. Nobel laureate Wendell Stanley remarked in 1970 that their 1944 announcement was an "undiscovered discovery." Stanley, however, was inexcusably wrong in this statement. No one knew better than he that Erwin Chargaff, the rather curmudgeon-like biochemist at Columbia University, on reading the Avery paper, had immediately stopped the chemical studies he had been doing and begun to concentrate on the chemical structure of DNA. He published in 1949 the first of his demonstrations that there was a one-to-one ratio between the purines and pyrimidines in the DNA molecule. Watson, Crick, and Wilkins later acknowledged the critical importance of this work in their approach to the structure of DNA.

The transcendent importance of the 1944 discovery can be easily recognized when one remembers, as James Watson relates in *The Double Helix*, that it was the demonstration that DNA was a hereditary-bearing molecule that led to Watson and Crick's decision in 1951 to study its molecular structure.

So, less than ten years after this seminal publication, the structure of DNA and its genetic functions were discovered. This is not a long delay for a major accomplishment, as we see when we contrast the forty-two-year interval between the origin of tissue culture and the actual administration of polio vaccine.

Whenever we recall our visits with Maurice Wilkins, almost reflexly these two lines from John Keats arise in our memory:

> Ay, in the very temple of Delight
> Veiled Melancholy has her sovran shrine.

We are not sure why these lines bubble into our consciousness as soon as we think of this great scientist. Perhaps it is because we immediately remember the devastating sadness Wilkins suffered for so many of his younger years because of the chronic, progressive illness that crippled his sister. Then too, in 1953, he experienced what Sir Lawrence Bragg described as "just frightfully bad luck."[6] This experience will be described farther on. It seems more likely that we began to think of the Keatsian lines after Wilkins told us that it was not easy for him to be cheerful because he was "more at home with sadness."

But enough of this prefatory melancholia. There is a story to be told that Wilkins began and almost finished, a story of the final unraveling of the puzzle that had obscured the key to life — the molecular structure of DNA.

Napoleon would never have chosen the New Zealand–born, Anglo-Irish Maurice Wilkins as one of his marshals, even though Wilkins probably is a more insightful scientist than Napoleon was a strategist. Wilkins was endowed with some elegant gifts, but panache was not one of them. Essentially reserved; possessing a soft, moderately pitched, unhurried voice; having a face handsome but delicate, with its deep-set, light blue eyes and its straight, sharp nose, Wilkins appears to be precisely what he is — an erudite, pensive scholar (see Fig. 9).

Our story begins in 1944–1945 with Wilkins in Berkeley, working on the Manhattan Project, unhappily isolating various uranium isotopes. He was probably lonely in the evenings, having recently been divorced from his young American wife. It was during one of these slow evenings that he perused Erwin Schrödinger's little book, *What Is Life?*[7]

Wilkins believes that it was reading this book that persuaded him to devote his career, once World War II had ended, to an investigation of the gene. He had read also of the discovery by Avery and his associates. Thus for Wilkins, as early as 1946, the book by Schrödinger plus the report by Avery equaled a revolutionary sum: DNA was the bearer of heredity.

It was fortunate for him that in 1947 he moved with his chief, the remarkable John Randall, to King's College in London. Randall not only served as chief of the Wheatstone physics department but also was able to wangle from the austere and quite conservative Medical Research Council (MRC) its financial subsidization of England's first biophysics laboratory. Prior to its establishment biologists, physicians, even biochemists considered physicists to be essentially of no value to medical research. Actually,

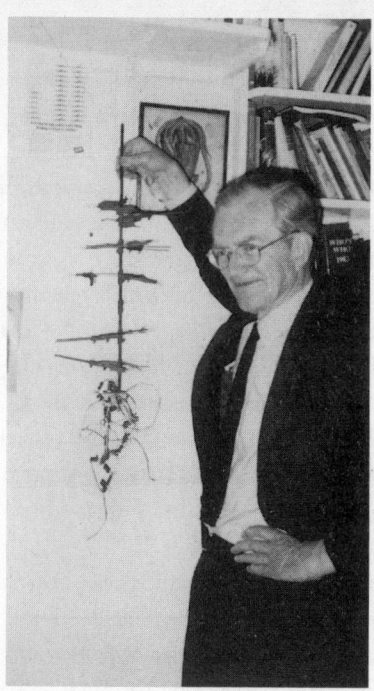

FIGURE 9. Maurice Wilkins in 1988,
holding a model of a unit of the DNA
macromolecular structure.

it is quite possible that the MRC members agreed to support Randall in this new venture not because they expected meaningful results, but because it was medicine's way of showing gratitude to Randall for saving England from destruction by the bombs of the Luftwaffe. They knew that the entire radar system depended on Randall's coinvention of its core component, the cavity magnetron.

So from 1947, Randall held down two jobs: running the King's College Department of Classical Physics and supervising the MRC-supported Biophysics Unit.

Maurice Wilkins, then a young man of thirty-one years, was asked by Randall to serve as assistant director of the Biophysics Unit. Randall, with much of the temperament of a Napoleon, liked to have as his subordinates scientists who were not only intelligent but also loyal. In Wilkins, whom he had known at Birmingham before the war and at Saint Andrews after the war, he had an ideal assistant. To Randall's credit, he knew of and was sympathetic to Wilkins' hunch that the study of DNA's structure was the correct course to take for an understanding of the genetic carrier.

Busy as Randall was directing two organizations, he still wished to tackle a research problem personally. He chose to investigate the physical structure of the bulbous head of sperm, where he knew its nucleoprotein was concentrated. He approached this problem through examination of the sperm's head by electron microscopy. In 1950 he asked Raymond Gosling, a graduate student working for his doctoral degree, to study the structure of the same sperm by X-ray crystallography. Gosling knew next to nothing about X-ray crystallography; but Alex Stokes, one of Randall's most talented physicists, knew quite a bit about submitting various chemical substances to X-rays. Randall asked him to instruct Gosling in this still-arcane physiocochemical discipline.

Although Gosling quickly mastered the basic principles of X-ray crystallography, he found that—given the dilapidated equipment at his disposal—he was not able to obtain satisfactory photo-diagrams of Randall's sperm heads. Somewhat in desperation he asked Wilkins for a bit of his DNA, in order to compare its X-ray diffraction photograph with the few diffraction photographs of sperm that he had succeeded in getting.

Wilkins had received a moderate amount of calf thymus DNA from a Swiss physicist. Rudolph Signer was so proud of the purity and physical integrity of his DNA that he brought samples of it to a London meeting of several scientists in May 1950. Wilkins was one of those who received the precious substance.

It was extraordinarily fortunate that Wilkins was given this meticulously extracted DNA. If he had not received this particular batch, the history of the discovery of DNA's structure would have been quite different. Unlike other samples of DNA that Wilkins had received, Signer's DNA made it possible for Wilkins to pick up single very thin, long fibers from the total gel-like DNA mass, merely by touching the mass with a clean glass rod.

Far more intrigued than Gosling to find out what sort of X-ray diffraction diagram DNA might yield, Wilkins agreed to give a thin fiber of his DNA to Gosling. Although the diffraction diagram Gosling obtained was a wretched mess, it did not prevent Wilkins from joining Gosling from then on in his study of DNA by X-ray crystallography. He was quite aware that W. T. Astbury as early as 1939 and S. Furberg as late as 1947 had employed this investigative tool to uncover some salient facts about the physical disposition of the molecules making up the huge macromolecule DNA. Indeed, Astbury had determined the distance (3.4 angstroms) separating the nucleotides of DNA, and Furberg had even hypothesized that DNA might have a helical structure.

It was Gosling who finally found a way to obtain a decent X-ray diagram of DNA: he gathered together thirty-five of Wilkins' finely drawn DNA fibers. Not only Wilkins was impressed, but also Stokes and probably Randall too. It could have been this first diffraction photograph that led Randall, in the spring of 1950, to recruit Rosalind Franklin on a three-year fellowship. Randall knew that she was a skilled, truly professional X-ray crystallographer; Wilkins and Gosling were at best intelligent amateurs in this elegant but somewhat exotic field. We shall hear much more about Franklin later on.

Unfortunately, in mid-1950, just as Gosling was getting fairly satisfactory diffraction diagrams for Wilkins and Stokes to analyze, the British Admiralty asked for the return of the X-ray machine it had only lent Randall. Wilkins was not too upset by this late-summer hiatus. He was reasonably certain that Gosling and he eventually could use an X-ray machine owned by another physics group at King's, but he was not happy with the necessity for X-raying bundles of DNA fibers. He recognized that if the group ever were to delineate the structure of DNA, it would have to obtain the X-ray diffraction diagram of a single DNA fiber, not a bundle of them. Therefore the X-ray beam would have to be markedly narrowed and the film-containing camera would have to be miniaturized.

Wilkins and Gosling were fortunate in that Werner Ehrenberg, a German refugee scientist, working with a colleague, Walter Spear, at Birkbeck College had just invented an X-ray device that they called a microfocus generating tube. This instrument was capable of concentrating diffuse X-ray beams to very narrow ones. It was just what Wilkins knew he had to have if he were ever to get a satisfactory diffraction diagram from X-raying a single tiny fiber of DNA. Gosling himself went to Birkbeck and Ehrenberg gave him this exceedingly precious instrument.

"It was truly important?" we asked Gosling forty years later.

"I believe," Gosling replied, "that it was an indispensable tool in our later X-raying of a single fiber. And guess what? This chap Ehrenberg wouldn't *sell* the microfocus tube, he insisted on giving it to us."

Wilkins realized that they would also need a microcamera, and he ordered one made by Phillips. So in the late autumn of 1950, they had the microfocus, the microcamera, and the borrowed X-ray apparatus of another physics unit. For some reason, neither Wilkins nor Gosling adapted the microfocus generator or the microcamera to the X-ray machine. It is probable that they expected Rosalind Franklin to come to the laboratory that same fall, in which case she could worry about the circuitry problems attendant on the installation of the microfocus tube and the optical niceties involved in employment of the microcamera. Franklin, however, delayed her arrival at King's College until January 1, 1951.

Wilkins by no means intended to withdraw from X-ray crystallography and occupy himself solely with his ultraviolet microscopic studies of DNA. He assumed that Franklin, a postdoctoral fellow, and Gosling would obtain the diffraction diagrams of single DNA fibers, then he and Stokes would analyze them. As the unit's pioneer in DNA research and as the assistant director of the MRC unit, he had every reason to expect Franklin's gracious and essentially subordinate collaboration. Wilkins was unaware of the fact that Randall, without consulting him, had written a letter to Franklin in December 1950 in which he stated that he wanted her to take charge of the X-ray crystallographic investigation of DNA. He also promised that Gosling would serve as her assistant. No one could have read this letter without assuming that she would work essentially as an independent investigator.

Wilkins also was unaware of the temperament of Rosalind Franklin. We might add that it also never occurred to him that John Randall was an ambitious, ruthless, no-holds-barred researcher himself. Randall undoubtedly recognized in the spring of 1950, when he first perused the X-ray diagrams taken by Gosling, the possibility that the discovery of DNA structure would far transcend in importance his coinvention of the cavity magnetron. Could he have planned to isolate Franklin from Wilkins, so that she would report her findings directly to him? If so, he again might be the senior coauthor (with her) of one of the century's most significant publications.

This possibility is not as far-fetched as it might at first glance appear. Randall had the reputation of running a tight ship, but he allowed the

Wilkins-Franklin feud to fester for two years without making it clear to Franklin that Wilkins was her immediate superior and that if she did not or could not report her findings to him, she would have to resign.

Wilkins himself, pondering decades later Randall's lack of communication about Franklin's place in the unit and his subsequent failure to deal decisively with her behavior, wondered if he had had an undetected research rival in John Randall.

Rosalind Franklin had an early appointment with death, and we believe she knew it early in her life. No sentient physician can peruse her studio photograph, which Francis Crick exhibits in his autobiography,[8] without detecting her deeply engraved sadness. Young women presenting this facial gloom *without* a contemporary cause more often than not may be unconsciously cognizant of their demise.

From her early teens Rosalind Franklin sought one thing from her cancer-shortened life: she ardently strove to be a respected scientist. Although she felt some affection for her family, as far as we know she felt no sexual passion for man or woman. Not at all tall, tennis slim, with jet black hair, deep-set brown-black eyes, and no makeup, Franklin was not pretty; she could have been stunning if she had chosen different clothes and brightened her face with cosmetics. But her goal was to become a topnotch scientist, not a party girl or a wife or a mother (see Figs. 10 and 11).

She was not altogether a pleasant person. Extraordinarily intelligent, she lacked the wisdom that gentleness of the heart and compassion of the soul sometimes create. All who knew her agreed that she did not suffer fools lightly. Tragically for both of them, she did not consider Maurice Wilkins a particularly bright man.

We have asked Wilkins, and also Francis Crick, James Watson, and Raymond Gosling, why Franklin as early as the spring of 1951 took a dislike to Wilkins. Ever since then, Wilkins himself has reflected on why neither could abide the other. He is writing his autobiography now, and we will allow him the courtesy of presenting his own answer. Neither Crick nor Watson was able to explain the cause of the conflict. Watson in *The Double Helix* tells of experiencing more than once her scorn and anger, but he treats her so pejoratively that he was advised to write an epilogue, which he did. In it he halfway apologizes for his bad-tempered treatment of this doomed but uniquely talented woman.

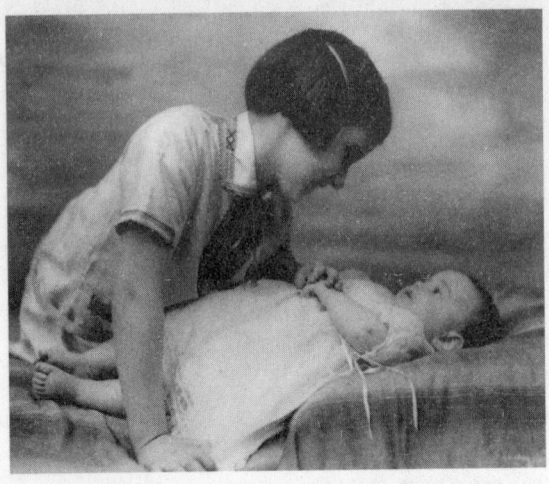

FIGURE 10. Rosalind Franklin at approximately ten years of age, caressing her infant sister, Jenifer. There is no hint here of the irascible, bad-tempered Rosalind described in James Watson's *Double Helix*.

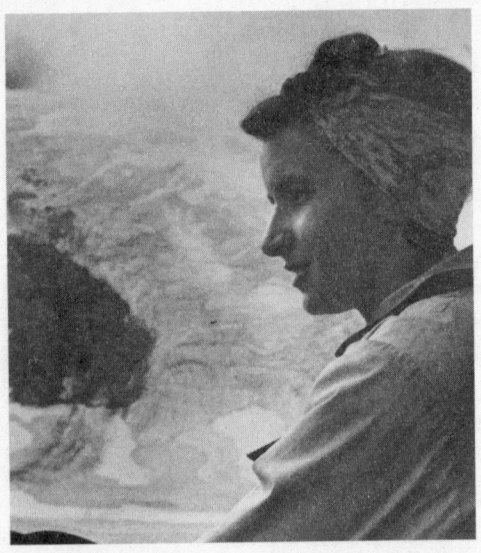

FIGURE 11. Rosalind Franklin during a hiking trip in the Alps when she was about twenty-eight years old. (Photograph by Vittorio Luzzati.)

We found Gosling to be the best source of information on the Franklin-Wilkins conflict, probably because he had the sensitive task of working with Franklin and still remaining friendly with Wilkins. This he managed to do, a feat that would astonish no one acquainted with Gosling's sincere charm. It came as no surprise to us that he liked both parties.

Gosling was absolutely certain of one fact: whether Franklin had been male or female, the antagonism would have occurred.

"They didn't get along from the very first. Maurice in those days was a sensitive sort of person, and Rosalind often had a tone of sarcasm in her voice when she criticized him. And she wasn't one bit hesitant about criticizing or arguing with him. I believe in those days Maurice expected women to exhibit deference and gentleness in their communication with their peers, and certainly with their superiors. Rosalind found it impossible to display either of those traits when she spoke or listened to Maurice."

"But you didn't find her difficult to get along with?" we asked.

"Not at all. You see, I was just a lowly graduate student, trying to get my doctorate."

"Did you ever sort of feel sorry for her?" we asked.

"Oh no, why should I have?"

We did not continue our questioning because Gosling suddenly exclaimed, "I just remembered something about Rosalind that I had paid no attention to. And it may have played a part in bringing on her ovarian cancer."

"What was that?" we asked.

"I remember her telling me that when she was working in Paris, on several occasions she was ordered to quit work for several weeks because her monitoring radiation badge indicated that she had been overexposed to radiation. She laughed when she told me about it because she thought it was ridiculous for her seniors to get exercised over what she considered nonsense."

"We gather that she did shield herself adequately when she worked at King's with your X-ray machine?" we inquired.

"No, she did not protect herself at King's, either. You see, she was intensely claustrophobic. During the air raids, she refused to enter any air raid shelter. But I'm not a physician, so I'm asking you if you think her

X-ray exposure could have played a part in her getting an ovarian cancer. After all she was only thirty-five when it began."

"It very well could have been responsible," we replied.

Open conflict between the two began in the spring of 1951, immediately after Wilkins had given a seminar at Cambridge on his and Gosling's X-ray diffraction studies of DNA. Rosalind, hearing of his talk, was furious. She approached Wilkins and in scathing, uncompromising terms told him that she and her student assistant, Gosling—not he—had been placed in charge of all X-ray studies of DNA. She ordered him to return to his ultraviolet microscopic studies of DNA.

Wilkins, in his own words, was staggered by this peremptory order from a "postdoc" fellow whom he had thought had been brought into the MRC unit to assist, or at least collaborate with, him; he was not only senior to her in years, but was assistant director of the entire Biophysics Unit.

Shocked as he was by her outbreak, he nevertheless determined that he and his colleague Alex Stokes would continue to take X-ray diffraction photographs of their Signer DNA fibers. Moreover this was precisely the time that he and Stokes were beginning to be quite sure that the DNA molecule had a *helical* conformation. Wilkins had just written a letter to Francis Crick to that effect and had even sketched a helix in the margin of his letter. Crick, at Cambridge, was not interested in DNA but in the protein molecule and thought Wilkins was wasting his time studying DNA. (This, of course, was before he met Watson later in 1951.)

Randall had been invited to give a talk in May 1951 at a physics conference in Naples, but at the last minute sent Wilkins in his place. When Wilkins gave his short talk on DNA, he showed a slide of a diffraction diagram that Gosling had obtained in mid-1950 when he exposed the bundle of Signer DNA fibers to his X-ray beams. A twenty-three-year-old "postdoc" fellow from Indiana, James Dewey Watson, happened to be in that Naples audience. Wilkins' talk did not particularly interest this bird-watching biologist, but when he saw Wilkins' X-ray diffraction slide he knew instantly that he might have found a way to answer the question that had nagged at him even before he had received his undergraduate degree: "How can I determine the nature of the entity that transmits man's hereditary messages to his offspring?"

Even before he saw Wilkins' crystallographic slide, Watson was positive that DNA was the macromolecule that carried these hereditary messages: the elegant publication of Avery and his colleagues had convinced him. He was sure that DNA was the carrier. To discover how this chemically simple macromolecule could execute such a complicated biological process, *that* was the challenge.

Watson's hunch lay in the hope—not the fact—that if he could lay bare the structure of DNA, it might reveal one of the basic mysteries of life, how a human passes on instructions to make another human. Seeing that single slide of Wilkins' gave Watson the tool he thought would supply the Nobel Prize answer to his question. Watson was not bothered for a second that he had no knowledge whatsoever of X-ray crystallography; he just had to find someone to teach him.

Watson related in his book that he schemed to meet Wilkins while the latter was still in Naples. Happening to see Wilkins the next day talking with his (Watson's) sister, Watson immediately began to daydream about encouraging Wilkins to fall in love and marry his attractive sibling. If that happened, he might be invited by Wilkins to join his staff.

The young American's daydream remained just that. Wilkins, after talking with Watson's sister as well as with Watson, apparently chose not to continue conversations with either. But Watson was determined to work with someone who could teach him the science, and the art, of X-ray crystallography. Having studied neither advanced chemistry nor physics, he was delighted that X-ray diffraction studies required only some expertise in mathematics. Watson did not have that expertise either, but was confident that he could acquire it.

Thanks to his former professor at Indiana University, he was accepted in the fall of 1951 at Cambridge's prestigious Cavendish Laboratory to work with the daunting biophysicist John Kendrew. Knowledgeable and skillful in X-ray diffraction techniques, Kendrew was using this tool to study the structure of hemoglobin and myoglobin. Apparently by mutual consent, Watson did not long assist Kendrew, and was left to do whatever he wished to do. The English biophysicists and biochemists making up the Cavendish staff probably were somewhat amused by this American visitor who, as Crick later wrote, perhaps "was too bright to be really sound." [9]

It just happened that Francis Crick himself (see Fig. 12) was thought to be too bright by most of the Cavendish staff, including its director, Sir

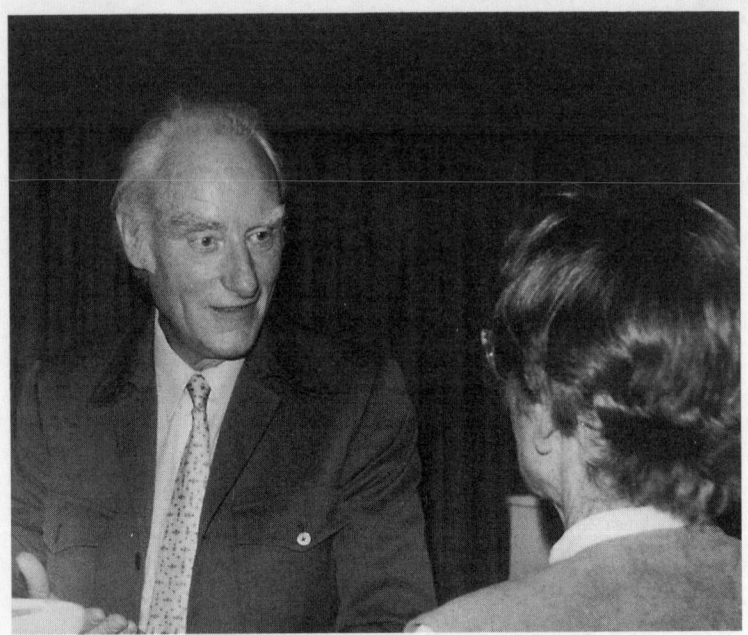

FIGURE 12. Francis Crick at a 1982 party, talking to his hostess, Dr. Macia Campbell Friedman.

Lawrence Bragg (who with his father had developed von Laue's X-ray diffraction into the science of X-ray crystallography).

Crick, thirteen years older than Watson, was working for his doctorate in biophysics. Although Watson considered himself a genius—an opinion with which we differ—few (or none) at the Cavendish agreed. However, the Cavendish group, even in 1951, knew that Crick too was very bright. He was so often critical of his peers and superiors, though, that he was not overly popular with any of the Cavendish scientists. We believe that Watson in *The Double Helix* exaggerated Crick's verbal obtrusiveness and the somewhat irritating quality of his laugh. We have met Crick on several social and professional occasions and were impressed with his capacity to listen to others. Nor did his laughter irritate us or our guests.

Neither Watson nor Crick describes in his memoirs the particulars of their first encounter. It is probable that the extraordinarily gifted doctoral student, who knew a lot about X-ray diffraction techniques and who loved to instruct other scientists, was precisely the person onto whom Watson could fasten to learn about X-ray crystallography. Watson also knew with the certainty that his intellect provided that it was this unknown Englishman whom he needed if he were to realize his dreams of unmasking the structure of DNA, attaining the Nobel Prize, and winning the heart of the most beautiful girl in the world.

We have seen that when Watson first arrived at Cavendish, Crick was not particularly interested in studying the structure of DNA. So it is a tribute to Watson's infectious enthusiasm that within several months of his arrival at Cambridge he had succeeded in involving Crick in his efforts to unravel one of life's major mysteries—how life continues. Moreover, he accomplished this feat despite the fact that Maurice Wilkins had been pursuing the same goal for the past several years. English scientists, as Watson pointed out in *The Double Helix*, rarely intruded into a field already occupied by a fellow scientist. This custom should have been observed by Crick, because he and Wilkins were warm friends.

Besides having to persuade Crick to compete against Wilkins, Watson had to overcome the reluctance of the director of the Cavendish Laboratory. Sir Lawrence Bragg knew full well that competing with fellow scientists simply was not done, particularly when all were financially supported by England's Medical Research Council. This English nicety failed to deter the American Watson. No such gentlemanly code had ever existed in the United States.

How, then, did Watson succeed in recruiting Crick to be his colleague? Like all the Cavendish investigators, he recognized Crick's superb mind. But he also needed a close English friend, and he wanted Crick to be that friend. Crick, for his part, could not help being pleased by this unusual American lad who *initially* listened to Crick as if to a Delphic oracle.

Further, Linus Pauling had just announced his discovery of the helical structure of protein. He had employed small multicolored plastic balls (representing atoms and molecules), building possible models of the protein molecule until he found the correct one. This discovery by means of model building had fired Crick's interest. As a friend, he had heard Wilkins express his opinion that the structure of DNA was helical. Also, Crick had already discovered by means of X-ray crystallography the theoretical constructs of protein's alpha helix.

So when Crick met Watson and discovered that Watson also suspected that the DNA molecule was helical in nature and that model building *plus* X-ray diffraction scrutiny was the way to determine the molecular structure of DNA, he could not resist talking hour after hour, day after day, with the avidly listening Watson.

Finally, Watson succeeded in recruiting Crick as his friend and scientific partner because Bragg and the other members of the Cavendish not only encouraged the liaison of this brash young American and the overage doctoral student, but saw to it that they shared an office and were able to talk and draw figures on the blackboard for hours every day, without bothering the other serious-minded scientists of the most prestigious physics laboratory in the world. Perhaps never before in the history of science was such a great scientific discovery achieved with so much theoretical conversation and so little experimental activity.

Both Watson and Crick realized that model building alone would not uncover the secret of the DNA molecule. They would have to pursue X-ray diffraction studies of DNA, as Watson had recognized on first seeing Wilkins' DNA slide. They also would require the help of biochemists (although they may not have realized this need in the fall of 1951).

They benefited hugely from Crick's ongoing friendship with Wilkins. It was vis-à-vis this friendship that Watson and Crick were intermittently informed of the X-ray diffraction studies of Rosalind Franklin. We cannot remember having read of any other scientific friendship that proved of such inestimable value to one participant and of so little value to the other as this momentous association of Crick and Wilkins.

It is unclear what sort of affiliation existed between Wilkins and Crick and Watson in the fall of 1951 when Crick decided to work with Watson on building possible molecular models of DNA. Much later (in October 1993) we queried Wilkins on this subject; he responded that Crick had been his longtime friend, and it was only natural to discuss with him his own X-ray crystallographic studies of DNA, and later those of Rosalind Franklin. However, he did not realize that Crick and Watson were working together as a team. More than likely, Wilkins believed that neither the young American nor Crick would get very far with their assembling and reassembling of red, white, and blue plastic balls. Despite Pauling's almost unbelievable discovery of the structure of the protein molecule via this kindergarten-like technique, Wilkins eschewed their usefulness in his own search for the structure of DNA.

Watson, convinced of the usefulness of the plastic balls, and of wires and metal plates, knew that Crick and he also needed guidance and confirmation during their sallies into model building. So when he was told by Wilkins that Franklin was scheduled to report on her X-ray diffraction studies of DNA in November 1951, he asked if he might be invited. Wilkins assured him that he would be welcome.

Although Watson attended the lecture, he took no notes and incorrectly remembered the amount of water Franklin had calculated that the DNA molecule contained. Depending heavily on what he remembered of her X-ray crystallographic data, and overlooking the critical purine/pyrimidine data that Erwin Chargaff had published,[10] Crick and Watson hastily constructed a supposed replica of the DNA molecule. They proudly exhibited their DNA model to Wilkins, Gosling, and Franklin—who came up from London to inspect this presumed Nobel-worthy masterpiece. Rosalind Franklin in just a few minutes found that they had succeeded in erecting only a piece of junk, a catastrophe that could have been avoided if Watson had correctly recalled the water content of the molecule. It is probable that Franklin was at her sarcastic worst in pointing out the total uselessness of the model.

Crick and Watson, after this visit of the King's College group, were crestfallen. They immediately recognized that Franklin's devastating criticisms were justified. Even worse, Bragg a few days later, having heard of this humiliating error, demanded that the two men immediately cease their DNA model building. From the beginning he had felt that they should not intrude into Wilkins' area of research. He found the devastating disaster an appropriate time to call a halt to a travesty that had begun because neither Watson nor Crick had found much else to occupy their keen, restless minds.

Officially, Watson and Crick halted their study of DNA. Crick offered to send Wilkins the jigs he and Watson had devised to fabricate the metal pieces of their model, but Wilkins was reluctant to add model building to his X-ray crystallographic approach.

Perhaps, though, their mandated cessation of model building encouraged Wilkins throughout 1952 to inform Crick more extensively than before about his own DNA studies. After all, Crick was his old friend. Then too, Franklin's increasing reluctance to speak to Wilkins, much less inform him of the results of her X-ray diffraction experiments, left Wilkins with no knowledgeable colleague at King's with whom he could talk about DNA.

Perhaps Wilkins in 1952 was not fully aware that Crick and Watson had by no means given up the pursuit of their goal. While they did cease model building, they continued to discuss various facets of the DNA problem as vigorously as before. The news that no less distinguished a scientist than Pauling had turned his attention to the DNA molecule further stimulated their efforts. They particularly sought the friendship of Pauling's son, Peter, who was studying at Cambridge. They knew that he could serve as a monitor of his father's research activities.

When Franklin first began to work at King's College in 1951, according to her notebooks she believed (as Wilkins had for a full year before her arrival) that DNA had a helical structure. But two occurrences later led her to insist that the structure was not helical after all.

The first was her discovery that depending on its water content, the DNA molecule could exist in either a relatively dry or crystalline state (the A form) or a relatively moist state (the B form). Because the A form was far more like a true crystal than the rather amorphous B form, she incorrectly decided that the A conformation was the correct form to study. A totally committed physicist, at home chiefly with inanimate and nonbiological materials, she was not cogently aware of the fact that almost all biological molecules function not as dry-as-dust crystals but as somewhat moist, colloidal entities.

Accordingly, during most of 1952 she was not able to determine by X-ray diffraction scrutiny the exact structural details of this A form of DNA. Despite the nicety of her written notes, her crystallographic results were trivial in importance. Even worse, she was not able during this entire year to discern a helical molecular structure from the X-ray diffraction photograph she took of the A form of DNA.

The second reason for her scornful rejection of the proposal that the DNA molecule was helical was that Wilkins, together with his colleague Stokes, became increasingly more insistent that DNA did possess a helical structure.

This is a serious indictment to make, but given the known stubbornness of Rosalind Franklin and her increasing dislike of Wilkins, it is not an unreasonable statement. Moreover, sometime in the late spring of 1952, employing the microfocus tube and microcamera that Wilkins had obtained in 1950 and X-raying a DNA fiber that Wilkins had received from Signer, long before she came to King's College Franklin succeeded in getting a positively resplendent diffraction photograph of DNA in its moist (or B) configuration. This photograph, now famous as Photograph 51, Franklin did not show to Wilkins or anyone else in the department because it unmistakably disclosed, to even a novice student of X-ray diffraction analyses, the helical nature of the DNA molecule.

Not only did Franklin not reveal this diffraction proof of the helical nature of the B form of DNA, approximately three months later she circulated to members of the Biophysics Unit cards that she had bordered with dense black ink. The cards bore this announcement:

> It is with great regret that we have to announce the death, on Friday, 18th July, 1952, D.N.A. HELIX (crystalline). . . . It is hoped that Dr. M. H. F. Wilkins will speak in memory of the late HELIX.

In writing this cruel card, Franklin still was careful to point out that it was the crystalline or A form of DNA that did not appear to have a helical structure. For she already knew that the B form was unquestionably helical.

Wilkins, of course, was not pleased by the circulation of this "memorial" card. But several months later, a colloquium given by Franklin on her studies convinced him that the A form of DNA was not helical. If he had ever seen Photograph 51 of the B form, with its unambiguous demonstration of the helical nature of this form, he would have continued to believe that DNA was helical. Not seeing this diagram, Wilkins apparently lost much of his interest in studying DNA.

At the end of 1952 Randall finally acted to restore peace in his laboratory. He asked Franklin to leave and turn over all her accumulated data to Wilkins. This she did. Wilkins then saw Photograph 51 with its unmistakable message. He was stunned. If he had seen the print six months earlier when it was made, and if Franklin had been cooperative and communicative, the two of them could well have solved the mystery of DNA's molecular structure.

In January 1953 Wilkins made a serious mistake: He showed Photograph 51 to Watson. He probably made this error because he was unaware of three developments. First, he probably did not know that despite Bragg's order in late 1951, Crick and Watson had continued throughout 1952 to work on DNA. Second, because he had never been enthusiastic about the model-building approach to determining the structure, he did not realize how close Watson and Crick were in their model building to a solution of the problem. Finally, he was completely unaware of the fact that they had Randall's 1952 report to the Medical Research Council, which carried certain data concerning the DNA observations of both Franklin and Wilkins. These data, added to Watson's instant recognition of the helix he saw in X-ray print 51, permitted Crick and Watson to finish correctly their construction of the DNA molecule.

The awesome and beautiful molecular structure they conjured up had a helix consisting of two chains that were bound together in some way by the purines and pyrimidines in the chains. Armed with this almost-complete molecular solution and the just-published but erroneous DNA molecular structure of Linus Pauling, Watson went to see Bragg in February 1953, asking his permission to work on DNA again.

He told Bragg how very close he was to solving the molecular structure of DNA, and that because Pauling was also attempting to unravel that structure, it now was an international competition between England and America, not just a family affair between the Wilkins group at King's College and the team at Cambridge. In short, Watson pleaded that they forget their previous trepidation about intruding into Wilkins' territory. Bragg, thus assailed and hating to let Pauling again beat him out, agreed that Watson could return to his model building. Of course, it must have been evident to Bragg that Watson already had been working on models. (In this conversation, Crick was not mentioned.)

Positive now that the DNA molecule had a double helical structure, Watson needed only to discover how the purines and pyrimidines of one chain linked up or bound to the purines and pyrimidines of the other chain. Throughout February 1953 he struggled with this problem. At first he attempted to construct models in which the two purines (guanine and adenine) and the two pyrimidines (cytosine and thymine) of one chain would combine with the analogous purines and pyrimidines of the second chain. This type of base pairing did not satisfy Crick, who was certain after seeing Franklin's data that the two chains ran in opposite directions. Nor did it satisfy the chemist Jerry Donohue, who pointed out to Watson on February 27, 1953, that he was using the wrong tautomeric forms of his bases, in that they should be in the keto rather than the enol form.

The next morning, employing cardboard replicas of the four bases, Watson stumbled on the correct way of connecting the two chains. When he joined guanine (a purine) not to another purine but to cytosine (a pyrimidine) and joined adenine (a purine) to thymine (a pyrimidine), the two chains fitted together marvelously. Thus, on February 28 Watson and Crick knew that for all practical purposes they had solved the structure of DNA. All that remained was to insert the metal plates representing the bases in the model and perhaps solder a few more wires representing hydrogen bonds. This they accomplished in the second week of March.

It was at precisely this time that Crick received the following letter from Wilkins:

My dear Francis,

Thank you for your letter on the polypeptides. I think you will be interested to know that our dark lady [i.e., Rosalind Franklin] leaves us next week and much of the 3 dimensional data is already in our hands. I am now reasonably clear of other commitments and have started up a general offensive on Nature's secret strongholds on all fronts: models, theoretical chemistry and interpretation of data, crystalline and comparative. At last the decks are clear and we can put all hands to the pumps!

It won't be long now.

Regards to all
Yours ever
M

Crick, after reading this letter, looked across the room where their completed model stood. Wilkins had cleared his decks to tackle a problem that already had been solved. Crick never answered this note. Apparently he asked John Kendrew, his senior in the laboratory, to notify Wilkins by telephone of their finished model.

Sometime before March 18, Wilkins received a copy of the manuscript Watson and Crick proposed to send to *Nature* for immediate publication.

Wilkins, on reading their manuscript, wrote Crick a letter whose first sentence was, "I think you're a couple of old rogues, but you may well have something." In the letter he suggested that his group, and also Franklin and Gosling, write articles that would be published together with the Watson-Crick article. Wilkins ended the letter with this sentence: "As one rat to another, good racing."

No one knows who managed it, but *Nature* reported that it received the DNA paper of Watson and Crick on April 3, 1953, exactly the same date on which it received the DNA report of Wilkins, Stokes, and Wilson and that of Franklin and Gosling. The articles were published together on April 25 under the general title "Molecular Structure of Nucleic Acids," with each of the three reports headed by a subtitle.[11] We believe this synchronization of publication was accomplished by agreement first between Bragg and Randall, then between them and the editor of *Nature*.

Not only were these reports of the Cambridge and King's College groups published simultaneously in *Nature*, they also were published together in a *single* offprint, something never done before. (Watson in 1993 stated that his article with Crick had also appeared as a separate offprint — but this happened after the combined offprint had been published.)

When one peruses these three papers, one may well ask why the single-page, eight-hundred-word report of Watson and Crick received overwhelming acclaim for the discovery of the molecular structure of DNA, whereas the two other reports received almost complete neglect.[12]

Examination of the April 25 issue of *Nature* divulges that the Watson and Crick report precedes (if only by one page) those of Wilkins and Franklin, thus permitting Watson and Crick to refer to the other two reports as the "following communications." Conversely, Wilkins and Franklin were forced to cite the report of Watson and Crick as "the preceding communication." The unfortunate fact is that to have the content of one's own article preceded by the content of someone else's article is to lose the holy grail of science — priority. Moreover, both Wilkins and Franklin stated, albeit in roundabout fashion, that their results confirmed the integrity of the Watson and Crick model. Franklin and Gosling concluded their article by saying, "Our general ideas are not inconsistent with the model proposed by Watson and Crick in the preceding communication." Watson and Crick thereby obtained admitted priority for their discovery and were reluctantly given confirmation.

In addition to precedence in the journal and lukewarm confirmation by the other two groups, Watson and Crick described their great discovery, that the twin helical chains are held together by purines binding to pyrimidines, in lucid, well-polished English prose with no pleonastic distraction. In glaring contrast, the papers of Wilkins and Franklin abounded in arcane jargon; it was as if they took joy in befuddling the reader with esoteric physicochemical data.

The truly magnificent coup de grace of Watson and Crick was the simple, hand-drawn diagram (by Crick's wife, Odile) of their proposed structure: two lines (representing two chains of molecules) curving about a vertical fiber axis, and separated by transverse lines representing the purine-pyrimidine base pairs connecting the two helical chains (see Fig. 13). Simple inspection of these curving chains made it easy to see that their separation probably was the mechanism by which all the cells of the body reproduced themselves.

After explaining the chemical constituents of these chains and the transverse bars separating yet connecting them, their paper contained the following sentence: "It has not escaped our notice that the specific pairing we have postulated immediately suggests a possible copying mechanism for the genetic material." This trenchant sentence, the contribution of Crick alone, did not escape the understanding of every scientist, regardless of field. In strong contrast, neither the poor delineation of the X-ray diffraction pattern in Wilkins' paper nor the striking diffraction illustration in Franklin's report could be expected to hold the attention of any scientist save a score or so of crystallographers. Fortunately for Wilkins, at least one of these crystallographers made it clear to the Nobel committee in 1962 how important these X-ray diffraction photographs were to elucidation of the molecule that determines every aspect of body and mind, and perhaps of soul.

Striking and provocative though this April 25 paper of Watson and Crick was, it was their second article in the same journal, just five weeks later, that proved to be their masterpiece of sheer intellection.[13] The first paragraph declared that these "many lines of evidence" indicated that DNA

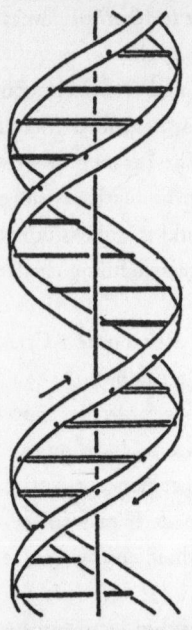

This figure is purely diagrammatic. The two ribbons symbolize the two phosphate—sugar chains, and the horizontal rods the pairs of bases holding the chains together. The vertical line marks the fibre axis

FIGURE 13. This figure, drawn by Odile Crick, and its accompanying caption appeared in the 1953 *Nature* article by Watson and Crick. (Reprinted by permission from *Nature* 171 [1953]: 737. Copyright © 1953, Macmillan Magazines Ltd.)

was the "carrier of a part of (if not all) the genetic specificity of the chromosome and thus of the gene itself." But there were no "many lines of evidence." There were only the data of Avery and his colleagues—which were not referred to in this report.

The article went on to say that their model for the structure of DNA had been given "quantitative support" by the X-ray evidence obtained by the King's College workers (meaning Wilkins and Franklin). Then Watson and Crick, having assumed that their model was confirmed by Wilkins and Franklin's *experimental* findings, felt courageous enough to state that their two chains were held together by adenine binding to thymine, and guanine to cytosine. This guess they bolstered by referring to Chargaff's *experimental* finding that in all the nucleic acids he analyzed the amounts of purine bases were essentially the same as the amounts of pyrimidine bases.

Having made these base-pairing assumptions, the authors pointed out that the DNA molecule was a long one, and any sequence of the base pairs could fit into the structure. Next, they made the awesome assumption that in a long molecule such as DNA with many possible base-pair sequences, "many different permutations are possible and it therefore seems likely that the precise sequence of the bases is the *code* which carries the genetical information."

Watson and Crick went on to say: "If the actual order of bases on one of the pairs of chains were given, one could write down the exact order of the bases on the other one, because of the specific pairing. Thus one chain is, as it were, the complement of the other and it is this feature which suggests how the deoxyribonucleic acid molecule might duplicate itself." They continued by stating, "Each chain acts as a template to itself of a new companion chain, so that eventually we shall have two pairs of chains, where we had only one before."

The authors, after modestly admitting that almost every statement in their article must be regarded as speculative and that much remained to be discovered, made this final declaration: "The hypothesis we are suggesting is that the template is the pattern of bases formed by one chain of the deoxyribonucleic acid and that the gene contains a complementary pair of such templates."

Sir Peter Medawar himself, one of England's most talented scientists, believed that this May 30 *Nature* paper of Watson's and Crick's was not only more important than his own Nobel Prize–winning discovery, but the most significant discovery of the twentieth century. He found the great thing about their discovery to be its completeness, its air of finality. He believed that if Watson and Crick "had been seen groping toward an answer" or if their solution "had come out piecemeal instead of in a blaze of understanding," the article would still have been considered well done "but not done in the grand romantic manner."

It bears noting that Medawar made these comments in 1968, fifteen years after Watson and Crick related their hypothesis. We seriously doubt that Medawar would have spoken in this manner in May 1953, when the second report appeared. He would have been inclined to believe that the entire hypothesis was a series of brilliant guesses, based solely upon the experimental findings of Avery, Chargaff, Wilkins, Franklin, and most important, the chemical aid of Donohue—who insisted that despite what Watson had read in textbooks, the purine bases in DNA were the keto, not the enol, form. It was this information from Donohue that led Watson to discover the bonding of the purines to the pyrimidines of DNA. For Wilkins already knew in 1950 that DNA probably had a double helical structure, and it was Franklin who first discovered that the bases of DNA formed the core of the DNA molecule; but neither Wilkins nor Franklin ever grasped the fact that adenine bonded only with thymine and guanine only with cytosine. This was the really amazing guess of Watson and Crick.

Never before had such a discovery been made by the simple combination of blackboard scrawling, absorption of the experimental work of others, perusal of other scientists' publications, and manipulation of plastic balls, wires, and metal plates. Not once in their several years of working together did either Watson or Crick touch or look directly at a fiber of DNA. They did not have to: Avery, Chargaff, Astbury, Wilkins, and Franklin already had done this part of the process for them.

Despite the informed and magisterial guessing of Watson and Crick in their May 30 article, as Crick later admitted there was no widespread or immediate acceptance of their daring hypothesis. However, in 1958 Matthew Meselson and Franklin Stahl performed an elegant experiment in which they employed density-gradient centrifugation after growing bacteria in a medium containing heavy nitrogen. They were able to confirm that DNA did possess a double chain that divided in the generation of the bacteria, with the subunits of each chain passing on to the daughter molecules, and that these original subunits were conserved intact through many bacterial duplications.[14]

Then Brenner and his colleagues uncovered the identity of messenger RNA, the molecule that carries messages from the DNA molecule to the ribosomes in the cytoplasm of the cell, and tells them how to synthesize one or more of the twenty amino acids. This last breakthrough was followed at the end of 1961 by Crick and Brenner's discovery of the general nature of the genetic code, an accomplishment that clarified and opened the field for all investigators interested in genetics.[15] These last two discoveries made it impossible for the Nobel committee to delay any longer in awarding the prize to Watson and Crick. And the committee did not forget Maurice Wilkins, the real pioneer of the enterprise. The three men were awarded the 1962 Nobel Prize in Physiology or Medicine.

The award process that year would have been very interesting had Rosalind Franklin not died in 1958. The prize cannot be given posthumously or shared by more than three persons. As already mentioned, Sir Aaron Klug believed she might have shared the prize if she had been alive in 1962. It must be remembered too that Crick, in a radio broadcast, freely admitted that without her help, Watson and he would not have arrived at their 1953 hypothesis. When we asked Watson, if Franklin had been alive in 1962, who then would have shared the Nobel Prize, he responded, without any hesitation, "Crick, myself, and Rosalind Franklin."

Despite these opinions of Klug, Crick, and Watson, it is our opinion that Wilkins deserved his share of the Nobel award as much or more than Watson and Crick. If there had been no Wilkins to first isolate a single fiber of DNA, to assemble the microfocus and microcamera as attachments to his X-ray machine, to inform Crick (as Watson reveals in *The Double Helix*) that the DNA molecule was too thick to represent just one chain of polynucleotides and so *the molecule was a compound helix of polynucleotide chains twisted about each other,* and all during 1952 to inform Crick of his own and Franklin's experimental data, there would have been no April 25 and May 30 *Nature* papers from Watson and Crick.

Today, forty-five years after publication of the three initial *Nature* reports, Watson has managed to obtain three positions (a professorship at Harvard, the directorship of Cold Spring Harbor, and for a while the directorship of the National Center for Human Genetic Research at the NIH), write and edit scientific monographs, and besides sharing the Nobel Prize, receive the Copley Award of the Royal Society and more than fifteen honorary doctorates (see Fig. 14). Now that he intends to write his autobiography, it will be interesting to see if his conscience finally has rid itself of the greeting given him by Willy Seeds in 1955: "How's honest Jim?" [16]

Crick, although offered honorary degrees after he shared the Nobel Prize in 1962, has resolutely refused all of them. After discovering the genetic code with Brenner, he ceased working entirely in genetics and began to study neurophysiology. He has held a chair at the Salk Institute for a

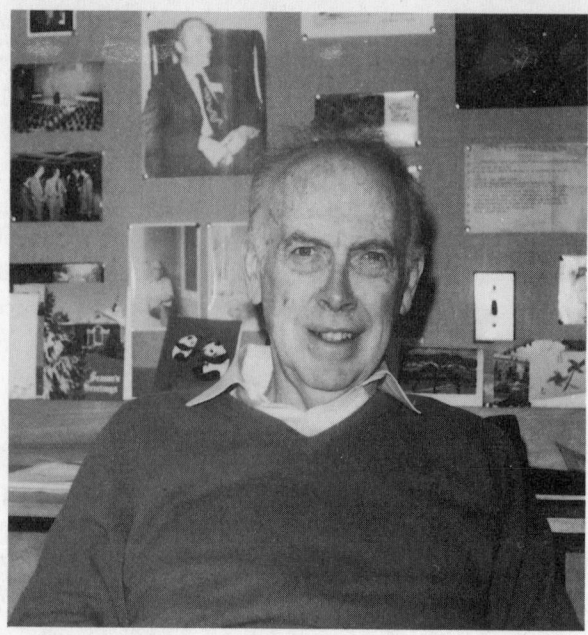

FIGURE 14. James Watson in his office in 1988. A newspaper
photograph of Francis Crick is pinned to the bulletin board.

number of years. From his desk he watches the sun-drenched Pacific Ocean
and mulls over the true function of dreams in our thought processes. Not
for a second does he agree with Freud's interpretation of dreams, even as
Freud would have sneered at Crick's book,[17] in which he propounds his hypothesis that life on earth began when a projectile sent from some other
planet crashed on earth and spilled the spores that eventually gave rise to
bacteria, amoeba, fishes, dinosaurs, and humans.

Wilkins has retired as a professor of molecular biophysics. For the first
several decades after his 1953 *Nature* article, he continued to accomplish distinguished X-ray diffraction studies of DNA and related molecules. Besides
sharing the Nobel Prize, he also received the Lasker Award. He remained
at King's College where, as an emeritus professor, he still gives lectures
to students at the college. He presently is working on his autobiography,
which will be as honest and as accurate as his eighty-one-year-old mem-

ory allows. He has had his difficulties writing this book, particularly in trying to present Rosalind Franklin at least as fairly as she may have deserved. And let us reemphasize that Maurice Wilkins has always been at a paradoxical sort of ease with sadness. Whenever we met with him, we were reminded of Yeats's observation, "Being Irish, he had an abiding sense of tragedy that sustained him in temporary periods of joy."

All of these matters we recalled one sunny afternoon in the fall of 1991 as we stared at the grave of Rosalind Franklin. The white marble walls of her sarcophagus gleamed in the bright sunlight, but the bronze letters affixed to the entablature already had eroded badly. Only after prolonged scrutiny were we able to decipher its brief message:

IN MEMORY OF ROSALIND ELSIE FRANKLIN

DEARLY LOVED ELDER DAUGHTER

OF ELLIS AND MURIEL FRANKLIN

25TH JULY, 1920–18TH APRIL, 1958

SCIENTIST

HER RESEARCHES AND DISCOVERIES OF

VIRUSES REMAIN OF LASTING BENEFIT

TO MANKIND.

Thus not even in death did Franklin receive credit for her contributions to the finest medical achievement of our century. But she *was* given credit for that which she wanted above all else, for being a scientist.

11

Concluding Thoughts

From the very beginning and throughout our selection of the ten magnificent achievements we have described, we found ourselves asking unanswered questions about these medical revelations. And we knew that at the end we would have to face and answer those haunting questions.

The obvious first question was, Which of these breakthrough achievements was the most important? We consulted professional colleagues, medical book collectors, and antiquarian medical book dealers. The two of us discussed this matter at length, after which we agreed to consider it separately and each make our own final decision. When we did so, we found we had both arrived at the same answer. We independently concluded that the single most important discovery of Western medicine was William Harvey's elucidation of the functions of the heart and the circulation of blood in the human body, because he had thereby introduced the principle of *experimentation* for the first time in medicine. He also recognized that the body and its parts moved, that life itself was a series of movements.

Our runner-up was the accurate description by Andreas Vesalius of the tissues and organs of the human body. At first, both of us were inclined to choose Vesalius' elucidation of the parts of the human body as our number one; but when we realized that Harvey's discovery initiated the field of physiology as we know it, we had to conclude that his finding that blood traveled in a circle had to be not only the greatest discovery of Western medicine but also the greatest medical achievement of all time.

The next question that had intrigued us from the very start was, What role did chance or luck play in these ten discoveries? Luck or chance was certainly responsible for four of them. If Antony Leeuwenhoek's rainwater had not happened to stand for several days in an open container, no bacteria would have proliferated in the water for him to discover with his microscope.

Similarly, Crawford Long would never have found ether as a superb anesthetic if one morning he had not remembered that the night before he had grievously bruised his limbs while enjoying an "ether party," strangely feeling no pain at the time he injured himself.

Who today could prophesy when X-rays would have been discovered if Wilhelm Roentgen had not, solely by chance, glanced at a tiny scrap of material lying, solely by chance, near his Crookes tube and detected its fluorescence?

Alexander Fleming's observation of the antibacterial action of penicillin would never have taken place if a tiny spore of *Penicillium* had not fallen into a petri dish that had been inoculated with, by chance, a bacterium that fortunately was susceptible to the inhibiting power of penicillin. But his discovery still would not have been made had he not taken a vacation at the precise time he did, and had a London heat wave not subsided at exactly the time the spore fell into the petri dish.

More than just chance was needed, however, before these four discoveries could be realized. They required patience, focus, and organization. And Leeuwenhoek, Long, Roentgen, and Fleming had these qualities in abundance.

Another question to be answered was, Did any of these ten discoveries evolve from another? The answer is yes! Certainly, if Vesalius had not discovered and described relatively accurately the constituents of the human body, Harvey seventy-five years later could not have made much sense of the heart as an integrated, functioning organ, and the network of arteries and veins would have been an impenetrable jungle of disparate vessels.

Again, if Leeuwenhoek and his followers had not revealed the existence of bacteria, Fleming of course would not have been aware of these organisms, much less interested in trying to prevent their growth.

These achievements were directly interrelated. But as we have already intimated, the eight great discoveries that chronologically followed that of Harvey would not have occurred if Harvey's revelations hadn't introduced the principle of *experimentation* in medical inquiry. For example, when one studies the findings of Jenner, Roentgen, Anichkov, or Wilkins, one discovers that experimentation played a predominant role.

Another question we asked ourselves was, Did these ten discoveries take place in any particular country or any particular societal or political ambience? The answers are equivocal.

Four of the ten disclosures occurred in Britain, two in America and in Holland, and one each in Germany and in Russia. Five of the ten were made in countries governed at the time by kings or emperors having almost absolute power. None of these rulers subsidized the initial researches leading to the great findings; but they subsequently honored or conferred financial gifts on the scientists who made the discoveries. The remaining five breakthroughs took place in democratic countries (Britain and America). Thus, it would appear that neither political absolutism nor democracy necessarily favors the appearance of great scientific observations—although, parenthetically, one of science's major discoveries (nuclear fission) was made in Hitler's Germany in 1939. Seven of the ten discoveries were accomplished in medical schools or universities; only the findings of Leeuwenhoek, Jenner, and Long were made in nonacademic environments.

If we turn now to our ten discoverers, we see that none was a genius as genius came to be defined from the late eighteenth century to the present. That is, none possessed that particular kind of intellectual power which has the appearance of proceeding from an *incomprehensible* inspiration and which seems to arrive at its results in an *inexplicable* and miraculous manner. For example, on reading the accomplishments of Harvey or Jenner, one is not as amazed at their results as one might be on hearing the Fifth Symphony of Beethoven, seeing the *Mona Lisa* of da Vinci or the *Pietà* of Michelangelo, or reading Max Planck's first description of quantum theory.

We admire the *natural*, totally understandable mental capacity of our ten discoverers. But we are not amazed at this mental talent, primarily because we can follow the working of their fine minds. Indeed, we almost believe that were we in their situations we might have arrived at their discoveries. None of us, though, has any illusion that we could equal the genius of Mozart's music, Shakespeare's dramas, or Newton's laws of physics. In short, our discoverers had ample talent but not genius.

If our ten heroes and their successors did not possess genius, all were endowed with not only an intense curiosity but, just as important, a capacity for methodical investigation of what evoked their curiosity.

Vesalius was almost obsessively curious about the bones of the human body, and he was the first scientist to realize fully that without the bones of our body, we would collapse to a soft blob of organs and tissues without any more mobility or function than a shell-less oyster. And without the external structural protection of the bones of our skulls, thought as we now know it would be impossible. Vesalius knew how to investigate this curiosity of bones methodically even if he had to fight in cemeteries after midnight against hungry wild dogs who were searching for human corpses to ravage.

Harvey's curiosity was extreme and broad. It was not confined to the heart, arteries, and veins. It was ignited also by the origin and function of megalithic Stonehenge, and he methodically attempted excavations at the base of the ancient stones. He was even more curious about the embryological development of various animals, a trait that led to his meticulous dissections of various species.

Leeuwenhoek was even more curious than Harvey. It was not only rainwater that he inspected with his microscope. He examined and described the tongue of a hog, the manure of horses, the lens of a whale, the eye of a flea. More important, he was curious about the content of his own blood, his own semen, even the scrapings of his own teeth.

As we already have described, Edward Jenner was equally curious about the underlying cause of angina pectoris as about the activities of the cuckoo nestling. Remember that he was not admitted to the Royal Society because of his discovery of vaccination, but because of his observations of the habits and the anatomy of the cuckoo nestling.

And what was it other than curiosity that drove Crawford Long to investigate ether, whose inhalation drove him to carouse enough to inflict injuries to his body yet protected him from perceiving any pain?

Nor would Roentgen have discovered the X-ray if he had not been curious about a small screen plated with barium platinocyanide and left a yard away from his Crookes tube, which began to emit greenish-yellow waves of light as soon as he sparked the tube.

If Ross Harrison had not been obsessively curious about how a nerve grows and lengthens itself, he would never have immersed a living nerve in lymph, thus inventing tissue culture.

It already was known that the yolk of an egg, when ingested by a rabbit or a guinea pig, led to atherosclerosis of the arteries of either animal. But it was Nikolai Anichkov's curiosity that made him seek out the chemical constituent of the yolk that was responsible for this malady.

Had Fleming not been a very curious man, after he returned from his vacation and noted that one of his culture plates contained not only bacteria but also a yellowish mold, he simply would have discarded the plate. But he *was* inquisitive about the impaired growth of the bacteria near the mold, and after methodical investigation he of course observed the antibiotic power of penicillin.

Maurice Wilkins is the only one of the ten discoverers whom we know personally. We have conversed with him for many hours, and he was kind enough to send us a draft of the first several chapters of his memoirs. While he is not as broadly curious a person as Jenner or Harvey must have been, he is curious enough to have inquired in considerable detail about not only our own scientific interests but also our families.

If these ten investigators varied a bit in the keenness of their talent or in the intensity of their curiosity, they did not vary in the degree of their persistence in making the observations and performing the experiments that led to their discoveries. Peculiarly, however, after they had made their discoveries, most of them turned to other activities: Vesalius after publication of the *Fabrica*, Roentgen after his discovery of the X-ray, and Fleming after his finding that penicillin was antibacterial.

Although all ten of our investigators married and most had children, it was their mistress whom they passionately loved. Without exception, this mistress was the hunt leading to their discovery. For her, wives and children, too, often suffered benign neglect. No son or daughter of our discoverers ever achieved even a modicum of distinction in any field of activity (although Nikolai Anichkov currently occupies his grandfather's position at the Medical Academy at Saint Petersburg).

Our ten researchers, with the possible exception of Harrison, sought fame as their reward. Vesalius in the half-dozen years before publication of the *Fabrica* in 1543 was driven by the desire to be recognized and accepted as one of the emperor's physicians, just as Fleming and Wilkins four centuries later were driven by their desire to win a Nobel Prize.

If our ten discoverers strove for recognition and fame, none lusted for money. Unfortunately, that is not the case today. Influenced by the money-seeking pharmaceutical companies, and more recently by even our most prestigious medical schools, too many scientific investigators want more than recognition. They also want to patent their discoveries to make money. If Roentgen were still alive, he would be shocked and saddened by the money orientation of our pharmaceutical companies and our universities. But in Roentgen's era, it did not require $200 million to finance the discovery and approval of a single medical drug.

Most of our ten discoverers were young (average age, 32.4 years) when they made their discoveries. Indeed, three (Vesalius, Long, and Anichkov) were in their twenties; Roentgen was the oldest (fifty years) at the time of his dazzling observation.

After we had described, as best we could, the scientific characteristics of our ten discoverers, we wondered which of them we would find the most interesting and, yes, charming to be with. We asked ourselves with which person would we be eager to spend a short (or even a long) vacation? Which person would be most likely to fascinate and charm the two mundane writers of this book with his interests and talents?

It was easy to eliminate eight of these men as vacation companions: Vesalius, because he was too cantankerous, too egotistical; Harvey, because he vastly preferred his own company and was not a congenial soul; Leeuwenhoek, because we have no idea of what he did besides looking at objects through his microscopes and selling dry goods; Roentgen, because he was an abominable speaker and had no interest in social matters; Harrison, because he was boring, even to Yale undergraduates, and socially austere; Anichkov, because in all the photographs we saw he looked grim, with no pleasing sparkle in his eyes; Fleming, because he was fundamentally downright boring; Wilkins, because he is too withdrawn and melancholy.

Both of us knew almost at once that it was Edward Jenner with whom we most desired to enjoy ourselves. If he vacationed with us and observed that we had no desire to hear about his marvelous experiments with cowpox, he would tell us about his discovery of coronary disease, or describe the lovable and not-so-lovable eccentricities of his beloved mentor, John Hunter. If we tired of these matters, he would tell us about the seasonal migration of English songbirds, as well as give further details about his beloved cuckoo. Seeing that we had heard enough of these trenchant observations, Jenner then might recite his own verses and get ready, at a minute's notice, to charm us with the lovely music he would create with his violin and flute. He would be happy to have us see, from the carriage drawn by two of his fine horses, his beloved Berkeley countryside. He would invite us to see Berkeley from the air, riding in one of the hydrogen balloons that he had invented. After these rides, he would warm us up with his best claret. Oh yes, we would enjoy such a time with Edward Jenner!

We wistfully wish we knew more about Crawford Long. The little we do know suggests that he too might be a delightful fellow vacationer. After all, it was his presence at a jovial ether party that led to his discovery of surgical anesthesia.

Even as we are finishing this book in the spring of 1998, Ian Wilmut has announced that he and his colleagues produced and raised a lamb who bears only her mother's genes. The cloned production of this animal is a momentous accomplishment. Its "inventor" would be the first to admit that his achievement depended on the discovery both of tissue culture and of DNA structure.

It is highly likely that sometime in the twenty-first century, a medical achievement will equal or even surpass the ten breakthroughs we have described in the preceding chapters. What might this discovery be? We believe that a series of experimental procedures eventually will lead to cures for those dread medical disorders, manic-depressive syndrome and schizophrenia. These two illnesses cripple and devastate the lives of millions of persons inhabiting our planet. Such a discovery probably will require tools and techniques not yet dreamed of; but we firmly believe they will be invented or found. Such an achievement will require the talents—and possibly the genius—of an investigator or team to whom the wonders of chemistry and physics are well known.

In the next century alone, the advances on all fronts of medicine will be a hundred times greater than all those of the last six centuries. The wondrous power given to medicine by the chemist, the physicist, and the engineer may well exceed the limits of today's imagination. It would be fascinating to know what the *next* ten major discoveries will be . . .

Notes

1. ANDREAS VESALIUS AND MODERN HUMAN ANATOMY

1. M. DeLuzzi, *Anothomia* (Pavia, Italy: Antonio De Carcano, 1478).

2. C. D. O'Malley, *Andreas Vesalius of Brussels* (Berkeley: University of California Press, 1964).

3. A. Vesalius, *Tabulae anatomicae sex* (Venice: J. S. Calcarenses, 1538).

4. Earlier, Leonardo da Vinci had executed wonderfully exact drawings of human tissues and organs, but they were not discovered until several centuries after his death. Even then, one of his drawings in the Royal Windsor Library, showing a human uterus and a vagina "sheathing" a fully erect male penis, was hidden from public view during the long lifetime of Queen Victoria.

5. A. Vesalius, *De humani corporis fabrica, libri septem* (Basel: Jounnis Oporini, 1543).

6. *Letter on the China Root*, 1546, translated by C. D. O'Malley as *Andreas Vesalius of Brussels* (Berkeley: University of California Press, 1964).

7. On page 662 of the *Fabrica* is sketched an unanesthetized, squealing pig. It is lying on its back, its extremities and upper jaw encased in chains that are secured to

a board, thus immobilizing the pig for dissection. A more hideous illustration would be hard to imagine. Certainly it was not drawn by John Stephanus of Calcar.

8. B. Eustachius, *Tabulae anatomica* (Rome: Gonzagae, 1714).

9. Eustachius pointed out that the kidney described and depicted in the *Fabrica* was that of a dog, not that of a human.

10. O'Malley, *Andreas Vesalius of Brussels.*

2. WILLIAM HARVEY AND THE CIRCULATION OF BLOOD

1. M. Servetus, *Christianismi restitutis* (Vienna: Balthasar Amoullet, 1553).

2. R. Colombo, *De re anatomica, libri XV* (Venice: Nicolai Beullacquae, 1559).

3. A. Cesalpino, *Peripateticarum questionum, libri quinque* (Venice: Apud Luntas, 1571).

4. G. Fabrici, *De venarum osteolis* (Padua: Lorenzo Pasquati, 1603).

5. W. Harvey, *Exercitationes de generatione animalium* (London: O. Pulleyn, 1651).

6. R. Lower, *Iractatus de corde* (London: J. Allestry, 1669).

7. M. Malpighi, *Opera omnia* (London: R. Scott, 1686).

3. ANTONY LEEUWENHOEK AND BACTERIA

1. Hooke, like Leeuwenhoek later, described the magnified appearance of objects that could be discerned by the naked eye (for instance, a duck feather, leaves, seeds, and the eye of a fly). In other words, Hooke presented some of the invisible details of visible objects. His *Micrographia* was one of the first books to carry the imprimatur of the Royal Society. The microscope employed by Hooke was a more complex instrument than that devised and constructed by Leeuwenhoek, but the lens ground by Leeuwenhoek was of much finer quality.

2. The entire letter was eventually translated from Dutch to English and published in 1932 by Clifford Dobell, a Fellow of the Royal Society, who authored the definitive biography of Leeuwenhoek: *Antony van Leeuwenhoek and His "Little Animals"* (London: John Bale, Sons, and Daniellson, Ltd., 1932).

3. W. Bullock, *The History of Bacteriology* (London: Oxford University Press, 1936).

4. L. Pasteur, "Thèses de physique et de chimie, presentées à la faculté des sciences de Paris" (Paris: Imprimeries de Bachelier, 1847).

5. R. Koch, "Die Aetiologie der Milzbrand—Krankheit, begrundet auf die Entwicklungsgeschichte des Bacillus Anthracis," *Beitrage Biologie der Pflanzen* 2 (1876):277.

6. R. Koch, "Die Aetiologie der Tuberkulose," *Berliner Klinische Wochenschrift* 19 (1882):221.

4. EDWARD JENNER AND VACCINATION

1. F. Fenner, D. A. Henderson, I. Arita, Z. Jezek, and I. D. Ladnyi, *Smallpox and Its Eradication* (Geneva: World Health Organization, 1988).

2. R. B. Fisher, *Edward Jenner, 1749–1823* (London: Andre Deutsch, 1991).

3. P. Razzel, *Edward Jenner's Cowpox Vaccine: The History of a Medical Myth* (Firle, England: Caliban Books, 1977).

4. J. Baron, *The Life of Edward Jenner*, vol. 1 (London: Henry Colburn, 1827).

5. I. Bailey, "Edward Jenner: Benefactor to Mankind," *Proceedings of the Royal College of Physicians of Edinburgh* 27 (1997):5.

6. T. D. Fosbroke, *Berkeley Manuscripts* (London: John, Nichols, 1821).

7. Fisher, *Edward Jenner*.

8. E. Jenner, "Observations on the Natural History of the Cuckoo," *Philosophical Transactions of the Royal Society* 78 (1788):219.

9. P. Saunders, *Edward Jenner, the Cheltenham Years, 1795–1823* (Hanover, N.H.: University Press of New England, 1982).

10. C. H. Parry, *An Inquiry into the Symptoms and Causes of the Syncope Anginosa* (Bath: R. Cruttwell, 1799).

11. Saunders, *Edward Jenner, the Cheltenham years*.

12. W. R. Le Fanu, *A Bio-Bibliography of Edward Jenner, 1749–1823* (London: Harvey and Blythe, 1951).

13. E. Jenner, *An Inquiry into the Cause and Effects of Variolae Vaccinae, a Disease Discovered in Some of the Western Counties of England, particularly Gloucestershire, and Known by the Name of Cowpox* (London: Sampson Low, 1798).

14. E. Jenner, *Further Observations on the Variolae Vaccinae or Cowpox* (London: Sampson Low, 1799); and idem, *A Continuation of the Facts and Observations Relative to the Variolae Vaccinae or Cowpox* (London: Sampson Low, 1800).

15. Fisher, *Edward Jenner*.

16. G. Miller, ed., *Letters of Edward Jenner and Other Documents Concerning the History of Vaccination from the Henry Barton Jacobs Collection in the William H. Welch Medical Library* (Baltimore: Johns Hopkins University Press, 1983).

5. CRAWFORD LONG AND SURGICAL ANESTHESIA

1. T. E. Keys, *The History of Surgical Anesthesia* (New York: Schumans, 1945).

2. M. Adt, P. Schumaker, and I. Muller, "The Role of Atropine in Antiquity and Anesthesia," in R. S. Atkinson and T. P. Boalton, eds., *The History of Anesthesia* (Carnforth, England: Parthenon, 1989), pp. 40–45; and J. F. Nunn, "Anesthesia in Ancient Times—Fact and Fable," in ibid., pp. 21–26.

3. U. Von Hitzenstern, "Anesthesia with Mandrake in the Tradition of Dioscorides and Its Role in Clinical Antiquity," in ibid., pp. 38–40.

4. M. T. Jasser, "Anesthesia in the History of Islamic Medicine," in ibid., pp. 48–51.

5. J. E. Echenhoff, *Anesthesia from Colonial Times: A History of Anesthesia at the University of Pennsylvania* (Philadelphia: J. B. Lippincott, 1966).

6. Keys, *The History of Surgical Anesthesia*.

7. Paracelsus, *Opera medico-chimica sive paradoxa* (Frankfurt, 1605), p. 125.

8. H. Davy, *Researches, Chemical and Philosophical, Chiefly Concerning Nitrous Oxide and Dephlogisticated Nitrous Air and Its Respiration* (London: Johnson, 1800).

9. W. P. C. Barton, "A Dissertation on the Chymical Properties and Exhilarating Effects of Nitrous Oxide Gas and Its Application to Pneumatick Medicine," M.D. thesis, University of Pennsylvania, 1808.

10. C. W. Long, "Account of the First Use of Sulphuric Ether by Inhalation as an Anesthesia in Surgical Operations," *Southern Medical and Surgical Journal* 5 (1849):705–713.

11. F. K. Boland, *The First Anesthetic: The Story of Crawford Long* (Athens: University of Georgia Press, 1950).

12. Ibid.

13. L. D. Vandam, "The Start of Modern Anesthesia," in Atkinson and Boulton, *The History of Anesthesia.*

14. K. B. Thomas, *The Development of Anesthetic Apparatus: A History Based on the Charles King Collection of the Association of Anesthetists of Great Britain and Ireland* (Oxford: Blackwell, 1975).

15. W. T. G. Morton, Circular, "Morton's Letheon" (Boston: Westworth, 1846).

16. Boland, *The First Anesthetic.*

17. H. J. Bigelow, "Insensibility during Surgical Operations Produced by Inhalation," *Boston Medical and Surgical Journal* 35 (1846):309, 379–382.

18. J. Snow, *On Chloroform and Other Anesthetics* (London: Churchill, 1858).

19. S. Guthrie, "New Mode of Preparing a Spiritous Solution of Chloric Ether," *American Journal of Scientific Arts* (1831):64–65; and R. W. Patterson, "The First Human Chloroformization," in Atkinson and Boulton, *The History of Anesthesia.*

20. W. Macewan, "Clinical Observations on the Introduction of Tracheal Tubes by the Mouth Instead of Performing Tracheotomy or Laryngotomy," *British Medical Journal* 3 (1880):122–124, 163–165.

21. F. Kuhn, *Die perorale Intubation* (Berlin: Karger, 1911); and G. M. Dorrance, "On the Treatment of Traumatic Injuries of the Lungs and Pleura with the Presentation of a New Intratracheal Tube for Use in Artification Respiration," *Surgery, Gynecology and Obstetrics* 2 (1910):160–189.

22. R. K. Calverley, "Intubation in Anesthesia," in Atkinson and Boulton, *The History of Anesthesia*, pp. 333–341.

23. J. W. Gale and R. M. Waters, "Closed Endobronchial Anesthesia in Thoracic Surgery: Preliminary Report," *Current Research, Anesthesia and Analgesia* 11 (1932):283–287.

24. J. A. Stiles et al., "Cyclopropane as Anesthetic Agent," *Current Research, Anesthesia and Analgesia* 13 (1934):56–60.

25. C. R. Stephen, C. M. Fabian, and L. W. Fabian, "Introduction of Halothane to the U.S.," in Atkinson and Boulton, *The History of Anesthesia*, pp. 221–222.

26. R. Hughes, "Development of Skeletal Muscle Relaxants from the Curare Arrow Poisons," in ibid., pp. 259–267.

27. H. Griffith and E. Johnson, "The Use of Curare in General Anesthesia," *Anesthesiology* 3 (1942):418–420.

28. E. Fischer and J. Mering, "Über eine neue Classe von Schlafmutheln," *Therape Gegenwart* 5 (1903):97–101.

29. J. B. Lundy, "Intravenous Anesthesia: Preliminary Report of the Use of Two New Barbiturates," *Proceedings of the Staff Meeting, Mayo Clinic* 10 (1930):536–543.

30. H. Braun, *Local Anesthesia, Its Scientific Basis and Practical Use,* 2d ed. (Philadelphia: Lea and Febiger, 1924).

31. W. S. Halsted, "Practical Comments on the Use and Abuse of Cocaine: Suggested by Its Invariably Successful Employment in More than a Thousand Minor Surgical Operations," *New York Medical Journal* 42 (1985):294–295.

32. J. L. Corning, "A Further Contribution on Local Medication of the Spinal Cord, with Cases," *Medical Record* 33 (1888):291–293.

33. A. Bier, "Versuche ueber Cocainisrung des Ruckenmarkes," *Deutsche zeitschrift für Chirurgie* 51 (1899):361–369.

34. A. Einhorn, "Ueber die Chemie der localen Anaesthetica," *Münchener Medizinischer Wochenschrift* 45 (1899):1218–20, 1254–56; and H. F. W. Braun, "Ueber einige neue orthohe Anaesthetica (Stovain, Alypin, Novocain)," *Deutsche Medizinische Wochenschrift* 32 (1904):1667–71.

6. WILHELM ROENTGEN AND THE X-RAY BEAM

1. O. Glasser, *Dr. W. C. Roentgen* (Springfield, Ill.: Thomas, 1958).

2. Crookes later was awarded the three most prestigious medals of the Royal Society (the Royal, Davy, and Copley medals) and in 1913 was elected president of the society. No other physicist has achieved all these honors.

3. R. L. Eisenberg, *Radiology, an Illustrated History* (St. Louis: Mosby Year Book, 1992).

4. P. Donizetti, *Shadow and Substance* (London: Pergamon, 1967).

5. W. Roentgen, "Eine neue Art von Strahlen" (Würzburg, 1895). This article appeared in the last ten pages of the 1895 volume of the *Proceedings of the Würzburg Physical-Medical Society.* A complete English translation, entitled "On a New Kind of X-Ray," can be found in Donizetti, *Shadow and Substance,* pp. 185–194.

6. B. H. Kevles, *Naked to the Bone: Medical Imaging in the Twentieth Century* (New Brunswick, N.J.: Rutgers University Press, 1997).

7. Glasser, *Dr. W. C. Roentgen.*

8. J. J. Cunningham and G. W. Friedland, "Early American Uroradiology, 1896–1933," *Urological Survey* 22 (1972):226.

9. G. N. Hounsfield, "Computerized Transverse Axial Scanning (Tomography). I. Description of a System," *British Journal of Radiology* 46 (1973):1016.

10. G. W. Friedland and B. D. Thurber, "The Birth of CT," *American Journal of Roentgenology* 167 (1996):1365.

11. A. M. Cormack, "Representation of a Function by Its Line Integrals with Some Radiological Applications," *Journal of Applied Physics* 35 (1964):2098.

7. ROSS HARRISON AND TISSUE CULTURE

1. J. S. Nicholas, "Ross Granville Harrison, 1870–1959: Biographical Memoirs," *National Academy of Science of the United States* 35 (1961):132–162.

2. R. G. Harrison, "Observations on the Living Developing Nerve Fiber," *Anatomical Record No. 5, American Journal of Anatomy* 7 (1907):No. 1.

3. R. G. Harrison, "On the Status and Significance of Tissue Culture," *Archiv für Zellforschung* 6 (1925):4.

4. Nicholas, "Ross Granville Harrison."

5. Letter, M. T. Burrows to Dr. Frederick M. Allen, New York, January 26, 1942. R. G. Harrison papers, Archives and Manuscript Departments, Sterling Library, Yale University, New Haven.

6. A. Carrel, "Rejuvenation of Cultures of Tissues," *Journal of the American Medical Association* 57 (1911):1611.

7. L. Hayflick, *How and Why We Age* (New York: Ballantine Books, 1994), pp. 127–142.

8. L. Hayflick, personal communication, 1996.

9. J. A. Witkowski, "Dr. Carrel's Immortal Cells," *Medical History* 24 (1980):129–142.

10. R. Buchabaum, personal communication, 1996.

11. Hayflick, *How and Why We Age*, pp. 111–136.

12. L. Hayflick and P. S. Moorhead, "The Serial Cultivation of Human Diploid Cell Strains," *Journal of Experimental Cell Research* 25 (1961):285–321.

13. M. A. Gold, *A Conspiracy of Cells: One Woman's Immortal Legacy and the Medical Scandal It Caused* (New York: State University of New York Press, 1986).

14. S. M. Gartler, "Apparent HeLa Cell Contamination of Human Heteroploid Cell Lines," *Nature* 217 (1968):750–751.

15. Gold, *A Conspiracy of Cells.*

16. W. A. Nelson-Rees, R. R. Flandermeyer, and P. K. Hawthorn, "Banded Marker Chromosomes as Indicators of Intraspecies Cellular Contamination," *Science* 184 (1974): 1093–96.

17. W. A. Nelson-Rees and P. R. Flandermeyer, "HeLa Cultures Defined," *Science* 191 (1976):96–98.

18. W. A. Nelson-Rees and P. R. Flandermeyer, "Inter- and Intra-Species Contamination of Human Breast Tumor Cell Lines HBC and Br ca5 and Other Cell Cultures," *Science* 195 (1977):1343–44.

19. P. Todd et al., "Comparison of the Effects of Various Cyclotron-Produced Fast Neutrons on the Reproduction Capacity of Cultured Human Kidney CT-D Cells," *International Journal of Radiation, Oncology, Biology and Physics* 4 (1978):1015–22.

20. Gold, *A Conspiracy of Cells.*

21. T. C. Hsu and C. M. Pomerat, "Mammalian Chromosomes *in vitro.* II. A

Method for Spreading the Chromosomes of Cells in Tissue Culture," *Journal of Heredity*, 44 (1953):23–29.

22. J. H. Tjio and A. Levan, "The Chromosome Number of Man," *Hereditas* 42 (1956):1–6.

23. R. G. Ham, "Survival and Growth Requirements of Nontransformed Cells," *Handbook of Experimental Pharmacology* 57 (1981):11–88.

24. A. B. Sabin and P. K. Olitsky, "Cultivation of Poliomyelitis Virus *in vitro* in Human Embryonic Nervous Tissue," *Proceedings of the Society of Experimental Biology* 34 (1936):357–359.

25. J. F. Enders, T. H. Weller, and F. C. Robbins, "Cultivation of the Lansing Strain of Poliomyelitis Virus in Cultures of Various Human Embryonic Tissues," *Science* 109 (1949):85–87.

26. Jonas E. Salk and associates, "Studies in Human Subjects on Active Immunization against Poliomyelitis. I. A Preliminary Report of Experiments in Progress," *Journal of the American Medical Association* 151 (1953):1081–98.

8. NIKOLAI ANICHKOV AND CHOLESTEROL

1. C. H. Parry, *An Inquiry into the Symptoms and Causes of the Syncope Anginosa, Commonly Called Angina Pectoris* (London: R. Cruttwell, 1799).

2. R. Virchow, *Phlogose und Thrombose in Gefass-system.* (Berlin: Gesammelte Abhandlungen für Wissenschaftlichen Medizin, 1856).

3. K. Rokitansky, "Ueber einiger der wichtigsten Krankheiten der Arterien," *Akademie der Wissenschaft Wien* 4 (1852):1.

4. F. Marchand, "Ueber Atherosclerosis," *Verhandlungen der Kongresse für Innere Medizin, 21 Kongresse,* 1904.

5. A. Windaus, "Ueber der Gehalt normaler und atheromatoser Aorten an Cholesterol und Cholesterinester," *Zeitschrift für Physiologische Chemie* 67 (1910):174.

6. A. I. Ignatowski, "Ueber die Wirkung der tiershen Einwesses auf der Aorta," *Virchows Archiv für Pathologische Anatomie* 198 (1909):248.

7. N. W. Stuckey, "On the Changes of the Rabbit Aorta under the Influence of Rich Animal Food," inaugural dissertation, Saint Petersburg, 1910.

8. S. Chalatov, "Ueber der Verhalten der Leber gegenüber den verschiedenen Arten von Speisfett," *Virchows Archiv* (1912):267.

9. N. Anichkov and S. Chalatov, "Ueber experimentelle Cholesterinsteatose: Ihre Bedeutung für die Enstehung einiger pathologischer Proessen," *Centrablatt für Allgemeine Pathologie und Pathologische Anatomie* 1 (1913):1.

10. A. Steiner and F. E. Kendall, "Atherosclerosis and Arteriosclerosis in Dogs following Ingestion of Cholesterol and Thiouracil," *Archives of Pathology* 42 (1946): 605.

11. C. H. Bailey, "Atheroma and Other Lesions Produced in Rabbits by Cholesterol Feeding," *Journal of Experimental Medicine* 23 (1961):69; and T. Leary, "Atherosclerosis,

the Important Form of Arteriosclerosis, a Metabolic Disease," *Journal of the American Medical Association* 105 (1935):495.

12. S. Weiss and G. R. Minot, "Nutrition in Relation to Arteriosclerosis," in E. V. Cowdry, ed., *Arteriosclerosis: A Survey of the Problem*, 1st ed. (New York: Macmillan, 1933).

13. J. W. Gofman et al., "The Role of Lipids and Lipoproteins in Atherosclerosis," *Science* 111 (1950):167.

14. L. W. Kinsell et al., "Dietary Modification of Serum Cholesterol and Phospholipid Levels," *Journal of Clinical Endocrinology* 12 (1952):909; and E. H. Ahrens, Jr., D. H. Blankenhorn, and T. T. Tsaltes, "Effect on Serum Lipids of Substituting Plant for Animal Fat in Diet," *Proceedings of the Society for Experimental Biology and Medicine* 86 (1952):872.

15. W. Dock, "Research in Arteriosclerosis—the First Fifty Years," editorial, *Annals of Internal Medicine* 49 (1958):699.

16. M. Friedman, R. H. Rosenman, and V. Carroll, "Changes in the Serum Cholesterol and Blood-Clotting Time in Men Subjected to Cyclic Variations of Occupational Stress," *Circulation* 17 (1958):852.

17. M. S. Brown and J. L. Goldstein, "Lipoprotein Receptors in the Liver," *Journal of Clinical Investigation* 72 (1983):743.

18. N. Anichkov, "A History of Experimentation on Arterial Atherosclerosis in Animals," in H. T. Blumenthal, ed., *Cowdry's Arteriosclerosis; A Survey of the Problem*, 2d ed. (Springfield, Ill.: Thomas, 1967).

9. ALEXANDER FLEMING AND ANTIBIOTICS

1. J. Tyndall, "The Optical Deportment of the Atmosphere in Relation to the Phenomena of Putrefaction and Infection," *Philosophical Transactions of the Royal Society* 166 (1876):27.

2. A. E. Duchesne, "Contribution à l'étude de la concurrence vitale chez les micro-organismes: Antagonisme entre les moissures et les microbes," dissertation, Army Medical Academy, Lyon, 1896.

3. D. Wilson, *In Search of Penicillin* (New York: Alfred A. Knopf, 1976).

4. R. Hare, *The Birth of Penicillin and the Disarming of Microbes* (London: George Allen and Unwin, 1970), chaps. 3 and 4.

5. A. Fleming, "On the Antibacterial Action of Cultures of Penicillium, with Special Reference to Their Use in Silation of *H influenzae*," *British Journal of Experimental Pathology* 10 (1929):226; and idem, "On the Specific Antibacterial Properties of Penicillin and Potassiuim Tellurite—Incorporating a Method of Demonstrating Some Bacterial Antagonisms," *Journal of Pathology and Bacteriology* 35 (1932):831.

6. Wilson, *In Search of Penicillin*.

7. A. Fleming and V. D. Alison, "Observations on a Bacteriolytic Substance ('Lysozyme') Found in Tissues and Secretions," *British Journal of Experimental Pathology* 3 (1922):252.

8. C. G. Paine, personal communication to Howard Florey, in H. W. Florey et al.,

eds., *Antibiotics — A Survey of Penicillin, Streptomycin and Other Antimicrobal Substances from Fungi, Actinomyces, and Plants* (London: Oxford University Press, 1949), p. 634.

9. P. W. Clutterback, R. Lovell, and H. Rainstrick, "Studies in the Biochemistry of Micro-organisms. XXVI. The Formation of Glucose by Members of *Penicillium chrysogenum* Series of a Pigment, an Alkali-Soluble Protein, and Penicillin — the Antibacterial Substance of Fleming," *Biochemistry Journal* 26 (1932):1907.

10. R. D. Reid, "Some Properties of Bacterial-Inhibitory Substance Produced by a Mold," *Journal of Bacteriology* 29 (1935):215.

11. G. Domagk, "Ein Beitrag zur Chemotherapie der bakteriellen Infektionen," *Deutscher medizinischer Wochenschrift* 61 (1935):250–253.

12. Wilson, *In Search of Penicillin.*

13. Ibid.

14. E. Chain et al., "Penicillin as a Chemotherapeutic Agent," *Lancet* 2 (1940):226.

15. E. P. Abraham et al., "Further Observations on Penicillin," *Lancet* 2 (1941):177.

16. G. L. Hobby, *Penicillin: Meeting the Challenge* (New Haven: Yale University Press, 1985).

17. R. J. Dubos, "Studies on a Bacterial Agent Extracted from a Soil Bacillus. I. Its Activity *in vitro*. II. Protective Effect of the Bacterial Agent against Experimental Pneumococcus Infections in Mice," *Journal of Experimental Medicine* 70 (1939):1.

18. A. Schatz, E. Bugie, and S. A. Waksman, "Streptomycin, a Substance Exhibiting Antibacterial Activity against Gram-Positive and Gram-Negative Bacteria," *Proceedings of the Society of Experimental Biology* 55 (1944):66.

19. R. Lewis, "The Rise of Antibiotic-Resistant Infections," *FDA Consumer* 29 (1995):11.

20. Data presented at a 1995 international meeting in Washington, D.C., on antibiotics and infections, organized by the *Lancet.*

10. MAURICE WILKINS AND DNA

1. J. F. Miescher, "Ueber die chemische Zusammensetzung der Eiterzellen," *Hoppe-Seyler Medicinisch-chemische Untersuchungen* 4 (1871):441.

2. R. Olby, *The Path to the Double Helix* (Seattle: University of Washington Press, 1974); F. H. Franklin and J. S. Cohen, *A Century of DNA: A History of the Discovery of the Structure and Function of the Genetic Substance* (Cambridge, Mass.: MIT Press, 1977); and H. F. Judson, *The Eighth Day of Creation* (New York: Simon and Schuster, 1979).

3. F. Griffith, "The Significance of Pneumococcal Types," *Journal of Hygiene* 27 (1928):113.

4. M. McCarty, *The Transforming Principle* (New York: W. W. Norton, 1985).

5. O. T. Avery, C. M. MacLeod, and M. McCarty, "Studies on the Chemical of the Substance Inducing Transformation of Pneumococcal Types," *Journal of Experimental Medicine* 79 (1944):137.

6. Judson, *The Eighth Day of Creation.*

7. Schrödinger, E., *What Is Life?* (Cambridge: Cambridge University Press, 1944).

8. F. H. C. Crick, *What Mad Pursuit* (New York: Basic Books, 1988).

9. Ibid.

10. E. Chargaff et al., "The Composition of the Deoxypentose Nucleic Acids of Thymus and Spleen," *Journal of Biological Chemistry* 177 (1949):405.

11. J. D. Watson and F. H. C. Crick, "Molecular Structure of Nucleic Acids. A Structure for Deoxyribose Nucleic Acid," *Nature* 171 (1953):737; M. H. F. Wilkins, A. R. Stokes, and H. R. Wilson, "Molecular Structure of Nucleic Acids. Molecular Structure of Deoxypentose Nucleic Acids," ibid., p. 738; R. F. Franklin and R. G. Gosling, "Molecular Structure of Nucleic Acids. Molecular Configuration in Sodium Thymonucleate," ibid., p. 740.

12. Fortunately, the 1962 Nobel committee did not overlook this report of Wilkins and his associates, or Wilkins' subsequent outstanding contributions. Nor did Sir Aaron Klug overlook Franklin's contribution; at the beginning of his Nobel acceptance lecture in 1982, referring to Rosalind Franklin, he said, "Had her life not been cut tragically short, she might well have stood in this place on an earlier occasion."

13. J. D. Watson and F. H. C. Crick, "Genetical Implications of the Structure of Deoxyribonucleic Acid," *Nature* 171 (1953):964–967.

14. M. S. Meselson and F. W. Stahl, "The Replication of DNA in Escherichia coli," *Proceedings of the National Academy of Science* 44 (1956):67.

15. S. Brenner, F. Jacob, and M. Meselson, "An Unstable Intermediate Carrying Information from Genes to Ribosomes for Protein Synthesis," *Nature* 190 (1960):576; and F. H. C. Crick et al., "General Nature of the Genetic Code for Proteins," *Nature* 192 (1961):1227.

16. This sarcastic salutation, as Watson relates in *The Double Helix*, was directed at him when Seeds, who had worked with Maurice Wilkins several years before, encountered Watson on an Alpine path. To Watson's surprise, after this greeting Seeds did not stop but walked away.

17. F. H. C. Crick, *Life Itself: Its Origin and Nature* (New York: Simon and Schuster, 1981).

Index

Anatomy (continued)

of, 16; *Tabulae anatomicae sex* by Vesalius, 5–6, 13; Vesalius's study of, 5–14, 17, 229–30, 231. *See also* Circulation of blood; *and specific organs of body*

Anesthesia: barbiturates, 112; chance in discovery of, 229; chloroform, 109–10; cocaine, 110, 113, 114; curare as muscle relaxant during, 112; cyclopropane, 111; dental anesthesia, 98, 102–4, 106, 107; divinyl ether, 111; epidural anesthesia, 114; epinephrine added to cocaine solution, 114; ether, 96, 98–101, 104–6, 114, 229; ethylene, 111; first use of term, 95; fundamental question on, 114; halothane, 111–12; injectable anesthetics, 112; local anesthetics, 112–14; nitrous oxide (laughing gas), 96–98, 103; novocaine, 114; obstetrical anesthesia, 100, 108–9; "pneumatic medicine," 96–98; side effects of and problems with, 109–10; spinal anesthesia, 114; Trilene, 111; Wells's role in discovery of, 102, 104, 105, 107. *See also* Surgical anesthesia

Aneurysm, 183–84

Anghera, Peter Martyr de, 112

Angina pectoris, 76–77, 92, 154, 231

Anichkov, Nikolai, 155–61, 165, 166, 167, 230, 232, 233, 234

Animal dissection. *See* Dissection

Animal research. *See specific animals*

Animal vivisection. *See* Vivisection of animals

Anthrax, 49–51, 55–56, 58, 64

Anthrax bacilli, 49–52, 55–56, 58, 169

Anthrax vaccine, 49–52, 55, 58

Antibiotics: Aureomycin, 190; Chain's research on, 178–82; chance in discovery of, 229; Chloramphenicol, 190; coinage of term, 190; cost of introduction of new drug, 190, 191; Domagk's research on, 177; Dreyer's research on, 177; and drug-resistant bacteria, 190–91; Fleming's research on, 170–76, 184–85, 230, 232; Florey's research on, 140, 176, 177–89; gramicidin as first antibiotic, 189; patent for penicillin, 184, 187–89; production and large-scale manufacturing of penicillin, 140, 182–89; Rainstrick's research on, 176; Reid's research on, 176–77; streptomycin, 190; Terramycin, 190; Tyndall's study of, 168–69, 171. *See also* Penicillin

Antirabies vaccine, 52–54, 55

Antitoxins, 60

Aorta, 32, 156, 157

Appendix, 169

Arabs, 66

Archaeology, 91

Argent, Dr., 29

Aristotle, 1

Arteries: and arteriosclerosis, 154–55; and atherosclerosis, 155, 156, 159, 165–67; and cholesterol, 154–55, 157; and circulation of blood, 19–20, 21, 29, 30–36; color of arterial blood, 36; coronary arteries, studies, 166; suture of cut ends of, 142, 145; Vesalius's description of, 13; X-ray examination of, 130

Arteriosclerosis, 154–55

Arteriosclerotic plaque, 154

Arthritis, 90

Aschoff, Ludwig, 157

Aselli, Caspare, 35

Astbury, W. T., 205, 224

Atherosclerosis, 155, 156, 159–60, 162, 164–67

Atherosclerotic plaque, 156–57